Practical Management of Spinal Injuries

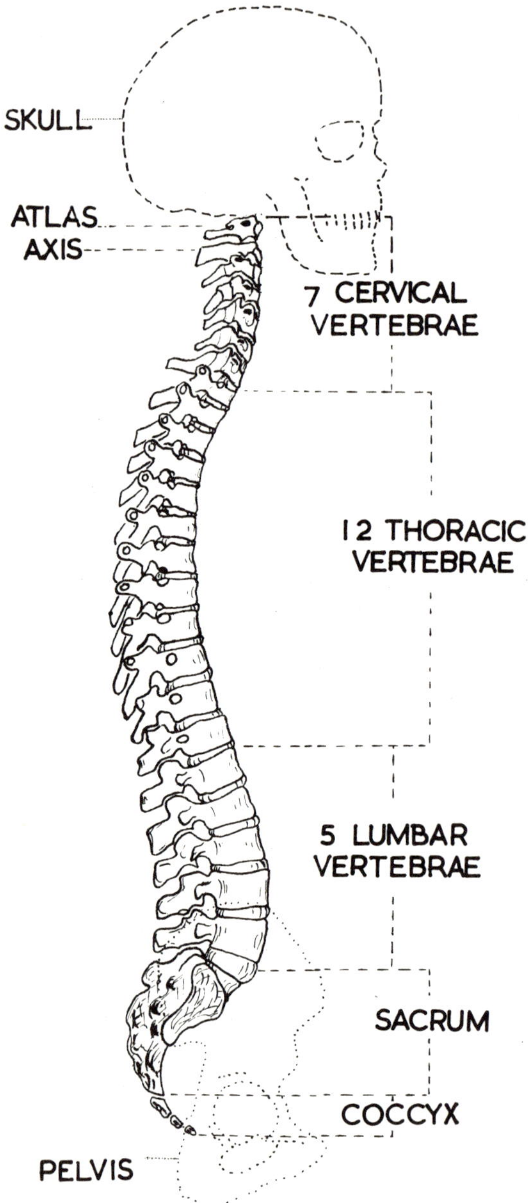

The human vertebral column.

Practical Management of Spinal Injuries

A Manual for Nurses

Alan G. Hardy
M.B.E., B.M., B. Ch. (Oxon), F.R.C.S. (Eng.)
Consultant in Charge, Spinal Injuries Unit,
Lodge Moor Hospital,
Sheffield

Reginald Elson
M.B., B. Ch., F.R.C.S. (Eng.)
Consultant Orthopaedic Surgeon,
The Northern General Hospital,
Sheffield

Foreword by
Sir Henry Osmond-Clarke
K.C.V.O., *C.B.E.*, F.R.C.S.
Former Orthopaedic Surgeon to Her Majesty Queen Elizabeth II;
Consulting Orthopaedic Surgeon, The London Hospital;
Consulting Orthopaedic Surgeon, The Robert Jones and
Agnes Hunt Orthopaedic Hospital, Oswestry;
Honorary Civilian Consultant in Orthopaedics, The Royal Air Force

SECOND EDITION

CHURCHILL LIVINGSTONE
Edinburgh London and New York 1976

CHURCHILL LIVINGSTONE
Medical Division of Longman Group Limited

Distributed in the United States of America by
Longman Inc., 72 Fifth Avenue, New York, N.Y.
10011 and by associated companies, branches and
representatives throughout the world.

First edition 1965
Second edition 1976

ISBN 0 443 01320 9

Library of Congress Cataloging in Publication Data

Hardy, Alan G
Practical management of spinal injuries for nurses

First ed. by R. Elson.
Includes index.
1. Spine—Wounds and injuries. 2. Orthopedic nursing.
I. Elson, Reginald, joint author. II. Elson,
Reginald. Practical management of spinal injuries for
nurses. III. Title. [DNLM: 1. Spinal injuries—
Nursing. WY161 H268P]
RD753.H37 1975 610.73'677 75-29262

Printed in Hong Kong

Foreword

Throughout history medicine has been beset with problems; for many centuries these have centred on the cure of established disease. Today the emphasis is on prevention of many of the diseases by which we were formerly afflicted, for example, skeletal tuberculosis and acute anterior poliomyelitis are almost unknown to the young doctors and nurses of the post World War Two generation.

But accidents—domestic, road and industrial—still produce formidable problems which seem likely to be with us indefinitely, in spite of the excellent research work carried out by the Medical Commission on Accident Prevention, inaugurated by Lord Porritt under the chairmanship of the late Norman Capener, now succeeded by Professor A. Harding Rains.

Of all the vast number of accidents throughout the world those that affect the spinal column and the spinal cord present in the survivors some of the most difficult problems in treatment and management—problems which involve the medical and paramedical disciplines, e.g. First Aid, nursing, physiotherapy, social workers, voluntary welfare bodies and so on.

In 1965 a wonderfully helpful monograph, *Practical Management of Spinal Injuries*, was written by Mr Reginald Elson, F.R.C.S. based on his experience in the Spinal Injuries Unit at the Robert Jones and Agnes Hunt Orthopaedic Hospital, Oswestry, which was instigated to serve the Midland Regions in 1955 by Professor Robert Roaf, and so successfully continued by Mr Terence McSweeney. In the second edition Mr Elson combined the authorship with Mr Alan G. Hardy, F.R.C.S. from the Spinal Injuries Unit, Lodge Moor Hospital, Sheffield whose vast and concentrated experience is in many respects similar to the pioneering work of Sir Ludwig Guttmann at Stoke Mandeville Hospital, Aylesbury.

This new edition emphasises even more than the first the difficult problems of visceral management and the importance of efficient nursing in the prevention of bed sores. With typical modesty the authors in their Preface maintain that the book is intended primarily 'for nurses specialising in the care of patients with spinal injuries'. So it is, but it should enjoy a much wider audience. In my view it should be a *vade mecum* for all lay and professional personnel dealing with these always difficult, and frequently formidable, injuries, for as the late Sir Reginald Watson-Jones wrote in the foreword to the first edition, quoting Mr Ernest Nicol, F.R.C.S.: 'Patients with paraplegia should be treated either superlatively well or not at all'. How true!

London, 1976

H. Osmond-Clarke

Preface

This book has been written for nurses specialising in the care of patients with spinal injuries. It is assumed that they have already gained working experience in general orthopaedic nursing.

It is difficult to gauge the amount of information which should be contained in a volume of this type. Although the basic principles are well established and unlikely to change, there are many controversial aspects. Another difficulty lies in the balance between medical and nursing care; while one consultant is prepared to allow nursing personnel to perform a particular duty or technique, another will be of the opinion that this is the task of a doctor. This book does not presume to dictate; suffice it to say that, in some institutions, the nursing staff are required to assume increased responsibilities in various ways. Accordingly, we have tried to indicate priorities and describe good techniques.

It is hoped that the book may prove of value to nursing staff who have been called upon to look after the occasional patient who, for some reason, has not been transferred to a spinal injuries centre; although written for nurses, it may be that doctors, physiotherapists and other experts in their own fields will find some points of interest herein.

The main differences between ordinary orthopaedic nursing and that required by patients with spinal injuries lie in the presence or absence of cord damage—before considering tetraplegia and paraplegia, injuries of the vertebral column have been described in order that the mechanisms responsible for the more serious conditions should be understood. It is for the purposes of description only that vertebral fractures and dislocations are dealt with separately from cord lesions; in practical management, bony, ligamentous and neurological damage comprise a single entity and must be treated as such. The brief section on disc lesions and minor back injuries has been included for the sake of completeness.

This presentation does not purport to present the *only* methods of treatment; there is immense scope for variation. All good centres have developed methods which in their hands give good results.

No attempt has been made to give detailed description of the management of very high spinal cord lesions. It is felt that these patients require treatment in super-specialised units where experience of respiratory and other problems can accumulate, as well as the availability of modern mechanico-medical devices. Probably one or two such centres should serve the whole of Great Britain until, as has been the case in lower lesions, more knowledge and experience is accrued.

A. G. H.
R. A. E.

Sheffield.
1976

Acknowledgements

The First Edition of this book was written in collaboration with many members of the staff of the Robert Jones and Agnes Hunt Orthopaedic Hospital at Oswestry. While much of the original text and illustrations are retained, many details have changed. The authors are grateful to Mr Brookes and Mr Martin for additional photographs, and to Sister Couldwell and Charge Nurse Crownshaw, Mr Goddard and Mr Charles, and the staff of the Spinal Injuries Unit of Lodge Moor Hospital, for making these possible. As always, patients have co-operated without exception in allowing themselves to be used as models.

A. G. H.
R. A. E.

Contents

Introduction

Accounts concerning the nature and management of vertebral injuries have appeared in medical literature for more than four thousand years; the uniqueness of spinal cord involvement has been well appreciated. The tragic loss of communication between two parts of the body which are, in themselves, healthy, has exercised a fascination for doctors and philosophers alike, and yet it is not until relatively recent times that we have been able to improve the lot of these unfortunate patients.

Most of the old writing on the subject described aspects of the vertebral and spinal cord injuries themselves; various methods of treatment of the injured parts were suggested in the hope that displacement of the bones might be corrected and resumption of cord function be achieved. Scant reference was made to what could be done for the victim should his spinal cord injury remain permanent.

It was during the First World War that the mass occurrence of this type of injury stimulated constructive interest in the situation, and much theoretical and practical study was performed; despite this, treatment compared with modern concepts was very poor. In the Second World War there was another wave of tetraplegic and paraplegic patients, and by this time there were men of vision who were able to show that by using modern methods of therapy and nursing, they could be taught a new way of life which, despite their affliction, was worthwhile and happy; no account of the management of spinal cord injuries must pass without tribute being paid to those who, with foresight and energy, tackled the seemingly hopeless and depressing subject of paraplegia and showed that it was wrong to regard these patients as 'better dead,' a hitherto common attitude. They showed the potential of good management so convincingly that new hope was found for the even greater task of improving the lot of patients with tetraplegia. It now appears that, given the right overall approach, patients having the highest lesions, compatible with life, can find some measure of happiness. It is not suggested that tetraplegia and paraplegia are to be regarded lightly, nor that management is easy—it is not; but because the mind has an immense facility for making the best of almost any circumstance, if the care is right in all respects, learning a new way of life is both possible and worthwhile. Without the right care, the statement made many years ago to the effect that cord injuries constituted 'an ailment not to be treated,' is probably justified.

Most of the war victims were healthy young adults. Now, another type of mishap is providing an increasing stream of spinal injuries—the road traffic accident. Domestic falls sustained by elderly people are also becoming more common; industry continues to contribute a fairly constant number of cases. There is a disproportionate increase in cervical lesions, some of which become tetraplegic; tetraplegia is the most serious consideration in this field because it demands such great aid for effective rehabilitation.

In England the patients with injury to the spinal cord are referred generally to one of the Spinal Injuries Units, and the pioneering work of Sir Ludwig Guttmann at Stoke Mandeville deserves the highest mention. Other units at Cardiff, Hexham, Oswestry, Pinderfields, Sheffield and Southport have also made contributions and any nurses wishing to study this subject should apply to visit one or more of the Centres and observe the programmes of overall treatment at first hand. The clear cut and decisive policies laid down by Sir Ludwig Guttmann will surely stand the test of time. Likewise in America the great work of the late Donald Munro and the now retired Dr Bors and Dr Comarr must receive special mention. The Veterans' Administration has provided facilities for the care of spinal cord injuries in a number of their hospitals throughout the length and breadth of the United States, and the pattern of these services is now being followed in Units established within civilian hospitals in some areas.

In 1964, the International Medical Society of Paraplegia was founded to co-ordinate, and report on, the work in the various Spinal Cord Injury Centres and to foster communication and co-operation on a world wide scale. The journal of the Society, which is called *Paraplegia*, reports on all aspects of spinal cord paralysis with a particular emphasis on trauma.

Sporting activities at local, national and international levels are now commonplace and the International Stoke Mandeville Games, which have been held annually, have a worldwide reputation.

The Disabled Living Foundation and the more recently formed Spinal Injuries Association furnish information about every facility and aid for the disabled, and details of all their services and equipment can be obtained from the respective headquarters, as well as through the Social Services Departments of the new local authorities. These services are designed to help patients to help themselves to achieve the highest degrees of compensatory physical independence within their capabilities. It is in this way that many patients can regain a life worth living, finding happiness in their home and interest in their local communities.

1. Vertebral Fractures and Dislocations

Usually, injury to the spine follows the forceful trauma of road traffic accidents, falls from a height and mishaps in heavy industry, e.g. mining; a special class of accident occurs in old people in whom the bones are weakened due to osteoporosis and deformed by degenerative osteoarthritis (especially cervical spondylosis). Injuries in warfare are commonly open wounds from gunshot or other missile, but civilian injuries are usually closed. Most of this account applies to the civilian type of injury; the incidence is rising steadily, especially in cases following road accidents.

It is necessary to have a clear understanding of the basic principles which underlie all aspects of management if these patients are to be nursed successfully.

The aims of management are:

1. To protect the spinal cord from injury, or to protect a spinal cord already injured from further damage
2. To aid healing of the injured vertebral column, thereby achieving stability and yet preserving mechanical function.

Anatomy

The vertebral column consists of a series of bones joined together by ligaments.

Each bone consists of a vertebral body on to the back of which is fixed a neural arch (Fig. 1.1).

Processes of bone protrude from the sides and posterior aspect of the neural arch which are levers on which the muscles controlling the vertebral column are attached. The range of movement between adjacent vertebrae is small, but because there are so many bones (seven in the cervical region, 12 in the thoracic region, five in the lumbar region; the last rests on the sacrum which is a solid bone), the total combined range of movement is considerable; the cervical part is the most mobile (Frontispiece).

The vertebral bodies are joined together by intervertebral discs which act as cushions and permit movement. These consist of a tough ring of ligamentous material uniting the outer part of the adjacent vertebral bodies, and this encloses a fluid cushion. The ring is called the annulus fibrosus and the fluid, the nucleus pulposus (Fig. 1.3).

The nucleus pulposus has been described as fluid, but with

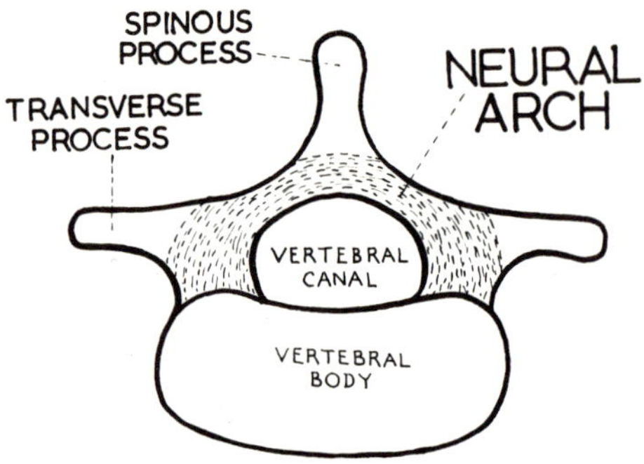

Fig. 1.1 The body and neural arch of a vertebra as seen from above.

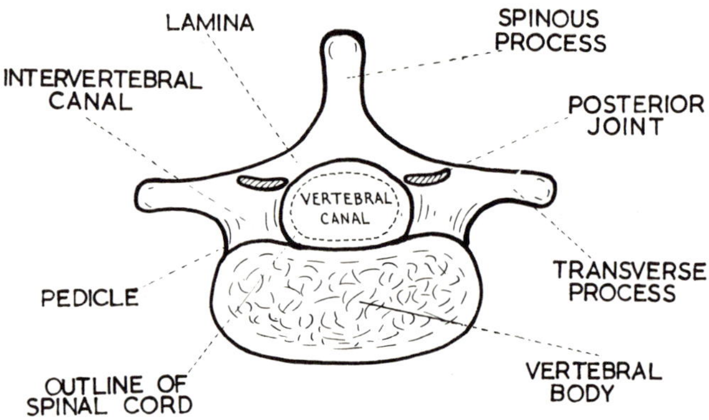

Fig. 1.2 The body and neural arch of a vertebra showing positions of the posterior joints and intervertebral canal.

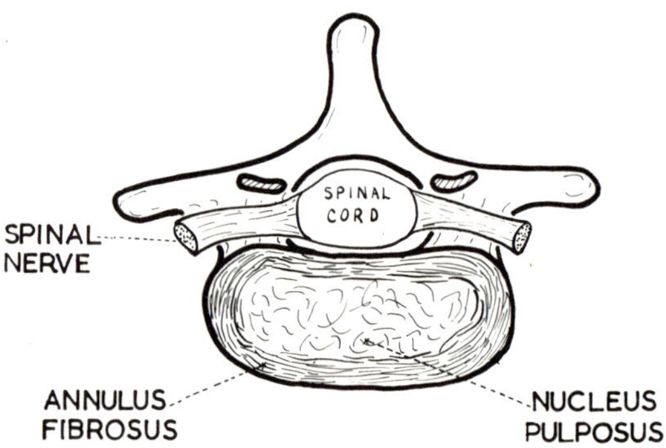

Fig. 1.3 Structure and position of the intervertebral disc.

increasing age it becomes progressively drier and ultimately, in the elderly, it is largely solid; this drying process is accompanied by a

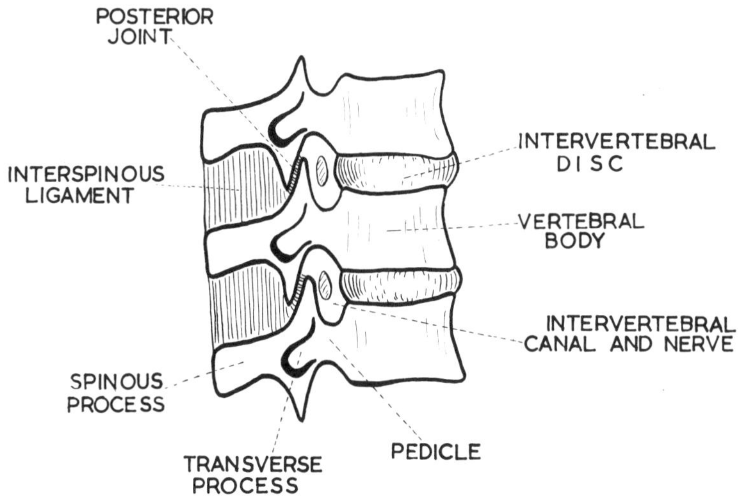

Fig. 1.4 Lateral view of three vertebrae showing the intervertebral discs (the anterior joint) and the posterior joints. Note the spinal nerves emerging from between these parts through the intervertebral canals.

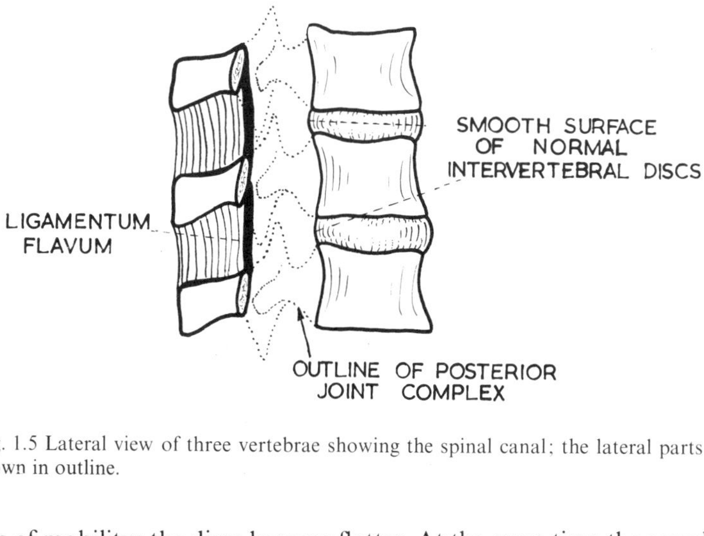

Fig. 1.5 Lateral view of three vertebrae showing the spinal canal; the lateral parts are shown in outline.

loss of mobility; the discs become flatter. At the same time the annulus becomes weaker.

Between the neural arches there is a synovial joint on each side (the posterior joints) (Fig. 1.2). The posterior part of the neural arches (the laminae) are joined together by elastic membranes called the ligamenta flava (Fig. 1.5). Other ligaments join the transverse processes and spinous processes. The ligaments which bind the bones together limit the range of movement between them, this range being normally controlled by the muscles. When distortion of the normal alignment is excessive, as may occur in violent accidents, the ligaments tear or, alternatively, pull off parts of the bones; the bones may be crushed in some types of violence.

The space enclosed by the neural arch is called the vertebral canal and it contains the spinal cord. Nerves escape from the vertebral canal through spaces between the front parts of the neural arch (Fig. 1.3) called the intervertebral foramina (singular: intervertebral foramen).

Other muscles are attached to the backs of the laminae, to both sides of the spinous processes and to the bodies themselves. The whole spinal apparatus forms a solid yet flexible and immensely strong column. Further control of movement is derived from the rib cage and abdominal musculature. Below, the column sits between the great bones of the pelvis, whence weight is transmitted to the lower limbs in the erect posture and to the ischial tuberosities when sitting. Above, the column supports the skull at the very mobile atlanto-occipital and atlanto-axial joints, where the bulk of nodding and shaking of the head occur respectively.

Unstable and stable vertebral injuries

When the spinal column is subjected to severe stress, the ligaments which join the vertebrae together may be sprained or ruptured, or the bones themselves may fracture. In some cases, following such an injury, a highly dangerous state can exist in which inexpert movement of the patient can cause further displacement at the site of damage, sufficient for the soft spinal cord to be squeezed between the bony fragments (Fig. 1.6). This type of injury is said to be *unstable*. In other cases, because mechanical linkage between fragments remains intact, further displacement cannot occur easily and the injury is said to be *stable*. The distinction between stable and unstable injuries is most important; without experience and exhaustive X-ray examination, it is not possible to say which state exists, and, because of this, the most important rule in the management of spinal injuries is: *all spinal injuries must be regarded as unstable until proved otherwise*. This rule applies in first-aid treatment, during transport, in Casualty and in the X-ray department. Even today occasional examples are seen of patients becoming paralysed from secondary cord damage while actually in hospital, because the rule was not followed.

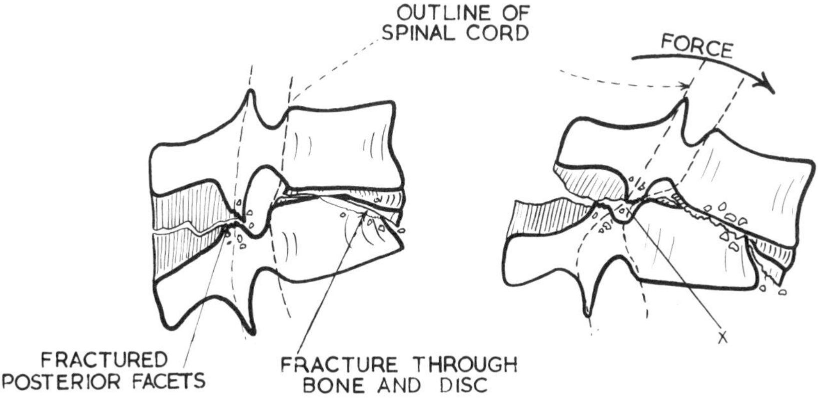

Fig. 1.6 Further displacement of an *unstable* fracture dislocation resulting in damage to the spinal cord. X marks the point of narrowing of the vertebral canal, a consequence of the further displacement.

The mechanisms of injury

The vertebral column may be subjected to a wide variety or combination of stresses. Because of the way we walk, stand, sit, crouch or travel, these stresses become grouped in the following ways: flexion, vertical compression, extension, lateral flexion, rotation—these forces are depicted on the whole human frame in Figure 1.7. Any level of

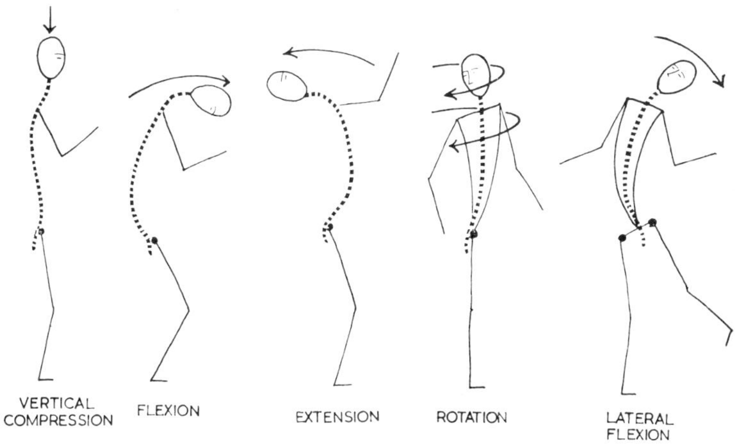

Fig. 1.7 A Pin-man being subjected to the various forces which can deform the vertebral column. Any part of the column can be primarily affected and any combination of the individual forces can occur.

the spinal column can be primarily affected. More specific examples will now be given.

1. *Flexion*

Examples. (a) A heavy blow across the shoulders or back of the head (Fig. 1.8); (b) A fall on to the heels or buttocks or on to the head from a height (Fig. 1.9).

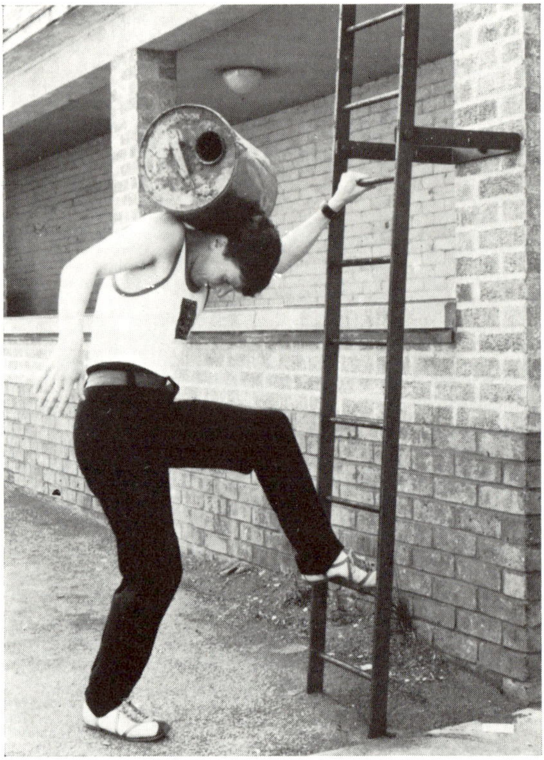

Fig. 1.8 Flexion injury of the cervical spine due to a blow on the head from a falling canister.

Results. In the *thoracic and lumbar* regions the vertebral bodies may become compressed and wedged; such a state is brought about by the bone crumbling and the resulting fine fragments becoming locked together (Fig. 1.10). Thus a wedge fracture is both comminuted and impacted. Provided the ligaments which bind the vertebrae together posteriorly remain untorn, and the neural arches are not fractured, these fractures are *stable*; if this is not the case, forward dislocation of one vertebra on another can occur and the injury is *unstable* (Fig. 1.11). In both cases a *kyphus* may be visible at the site of injury; the spinous processes may fracture.

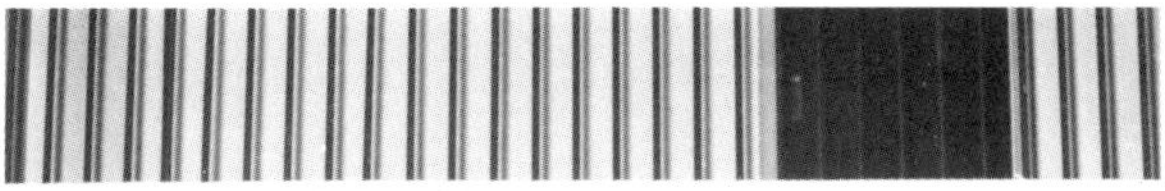

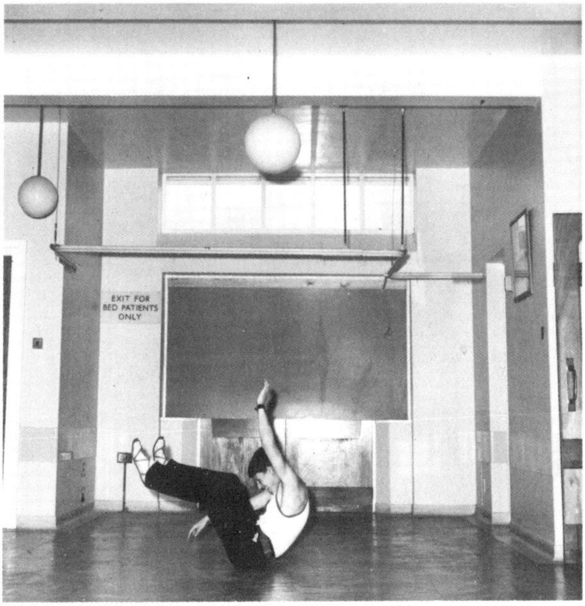

Fig. 1.9 Flexion injury of the thoracic and lumbar spines due to a fall on to the buttocks from a height.

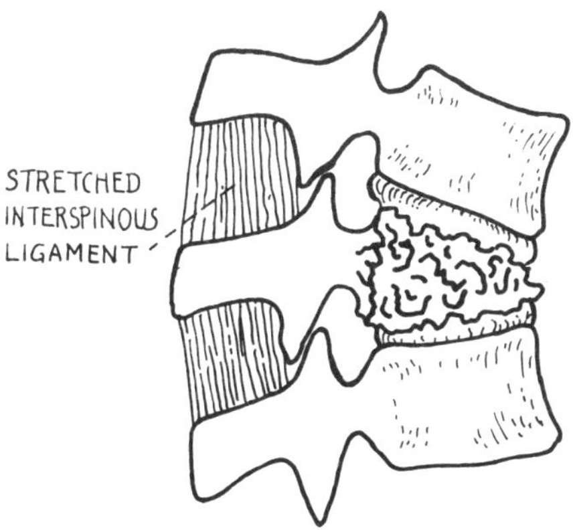

Fig. 1.10 A wedge fracture of the vertebral body.

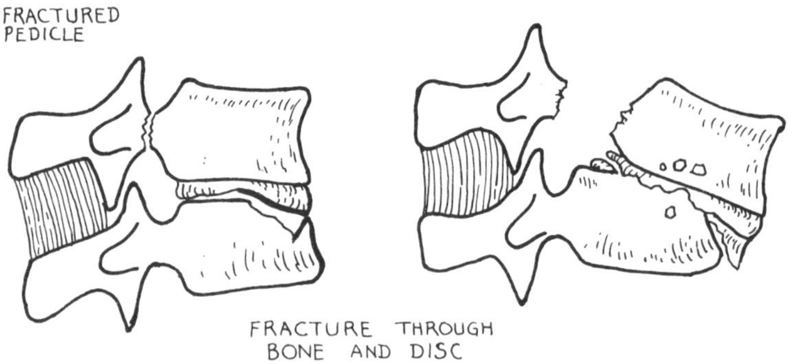

Fig. 1.11 Forward dislocation of one vertebra on another when posterior elements are ruptured; in this example the pedicles are fractured.

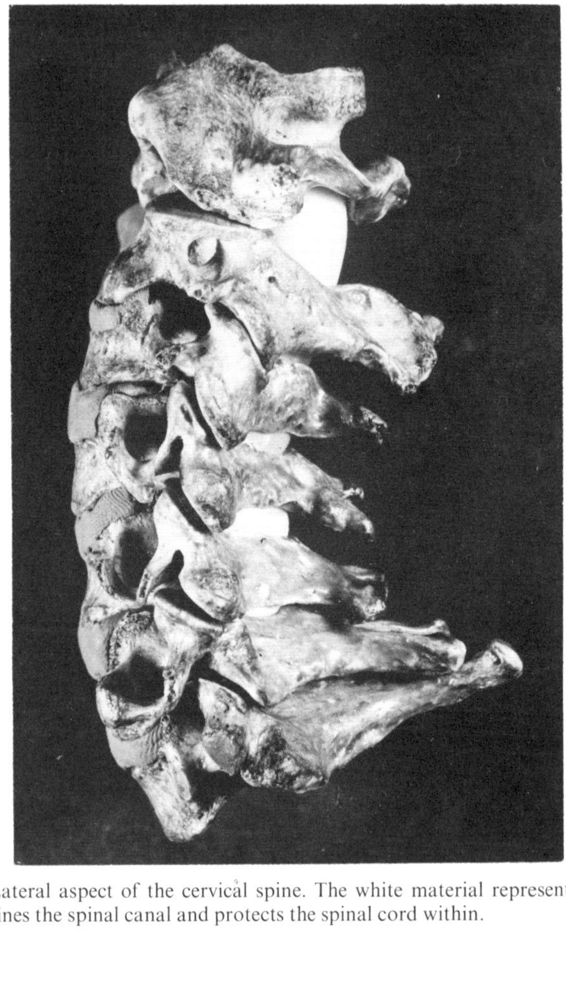

Fig. 1.12 Lateral aspect of the cervical spine. The white material represents the dural sac which lines the spinal canal and protects the spinal cord within.

In the *cervical* region, extensive ligamentous tearing may result in dislocation of one vertebra on another; such ligamentous damage may not be evident on X-ray because, following injury, the bones have slipped back into position, and yet a highly dangerous unstable situation exists. Sometimes the vertebrae can lock in the dislocated position (Figs. 1.12 and 1.13); sometimes only a subluxation occurs. Fractures through parts of the vertebrae may be present.

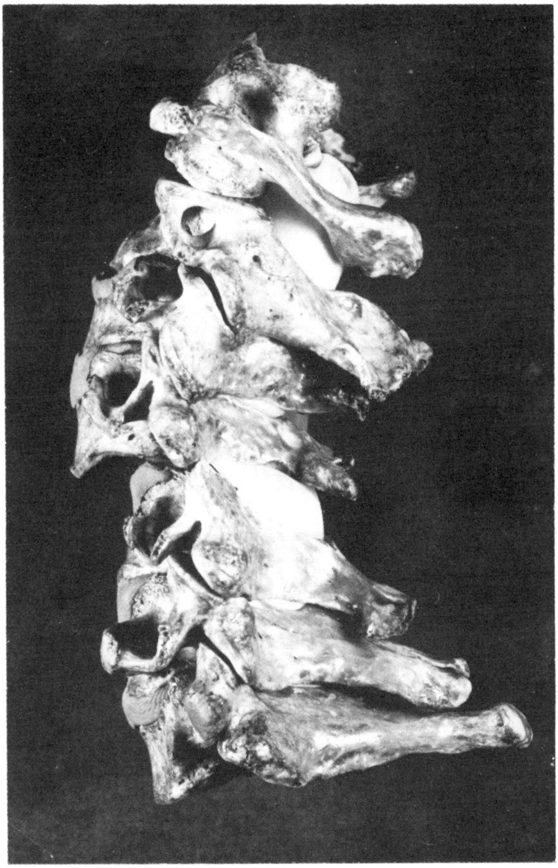

Fig. 1.13 Severely deformed dura, due to a forward dislocation of one vertebra on another.

2. *Flexion with rotation*

Examples. (a) A heavy blow on to one shoulder causing the trunk to be flexed forward and swivelled to the opposite side (Fig. 1.14); (b) a blow or fall on to the postero-lateral aspect of the head.

Results. Flexion with rotation constitutes a peculiarly potent combination of forces causing fracture-dislocation of the spine at any level, especially at the *thoraco-lumbar* region (tenth thoracic to first lumbar) and in the neck. One vertebra is twisted off the one beneath it, taking a slice of body with it. The body fractures and the disc remains partly intact. There is extensive damage to the posterior bony and ligamentous parts and this fracture-dislocation is highly unstable (Fig. 1.15).

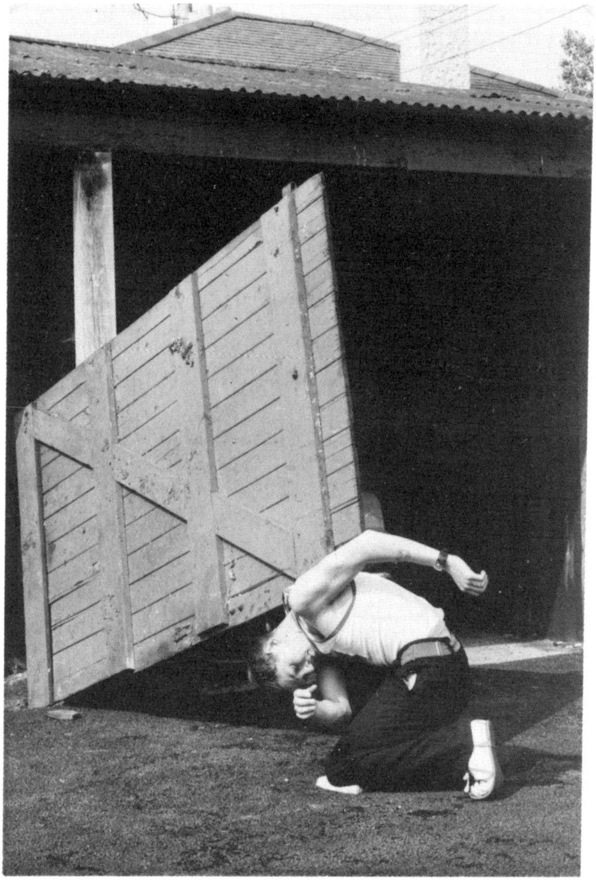

Fig. 1.14 Flexion rotation injury. The heavy door has fallen on to the subject's right shoulder so that his trunk is flexed and rotated to his left.

In the *cervical region,* dislocation of the posterior joint on one side only may occur.

3. *Vertical compression*

Examples. (a) A blow on the top of the head (Fig. 1.16); (b) a fall from a height in the erect position (Fig. 1.17).

Results. The bodies of one or more vertebrae are burst open; this

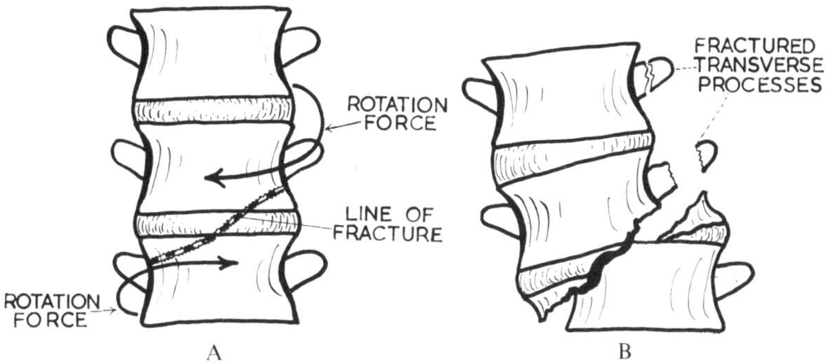

Fig. 1.15 A, The line of the fracture due to flexion rotation stress. Usually this fracture is seen in the thoraco-lumbar region. B, The sort of displacement which occurs in this 'slice fracture' due to flexion rotation stress. (*See* also Fig. 1.6.)

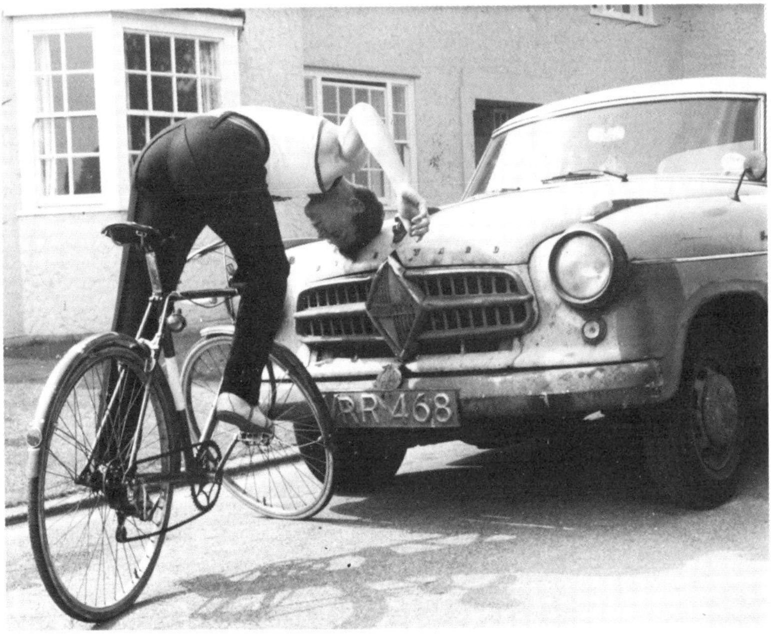

Fig. 1.16 A high velocity injury in which the cervical spine is subjected to vertical compression.

occurs because the compressed intervertebral disc is driven forcibly into the adjacent bone. Some disc material and bone may rupture into the vertebral canal and crush the spinal cord (Fig. 1.18). Frequently the shattering extends into the ring of the neural arch. This injury is *unstable*. It should be noted that, if there is time, the spine flexes when subjected to severe compression, but in injuries where the force has been applied very rapidly (high velocity injuries) the spine does

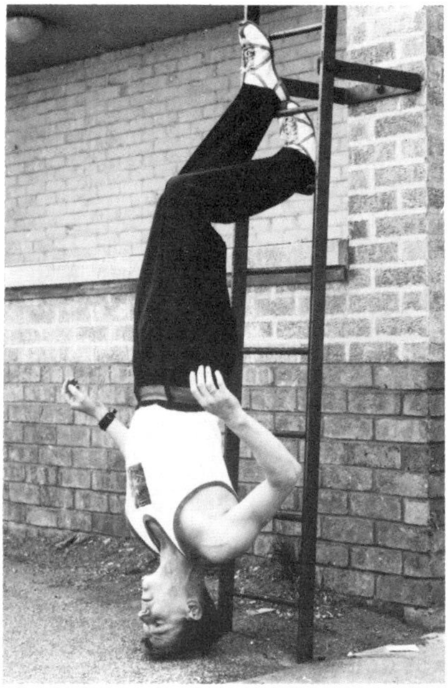

Fig. 1.17 Fall on to the head in the neutral position resulting in forceful vertical compression of the cervical spine.

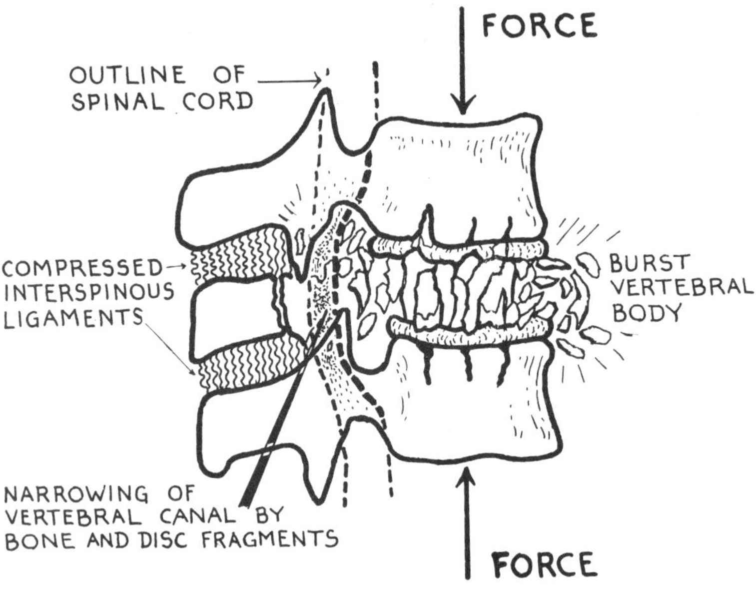

Fig. 1.18 The result of vertical compression, especially when this force is applied at high velocity. The shattered body bursts into the spinal canal.

not have time to react into flexion, but stays fully extended so that the purely vertical compression force is applied; it is in this way that a bursting fracture occurs and it is seen in many high velocity road accidents. It is most common in the *cervical* region.

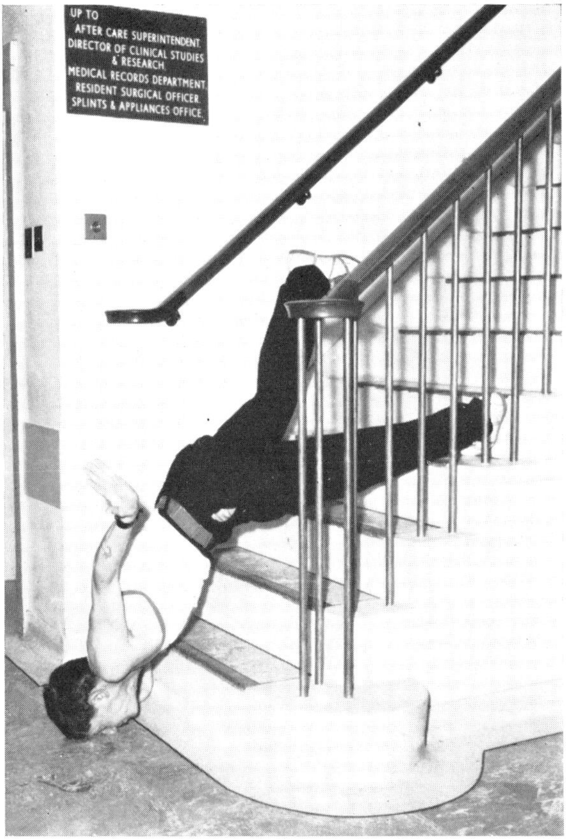

Fig. 1.19 A typical cause of hyperextension injury to the cervical spine, more usually seen in elderly people.

4. *Extension*

Example. A fall downstairs in which the forehead is struck and the head is jerked backwards, i.e. hyperextended (Fig. 1.19).

Results. Extension injuries usually involve the *cervical* spine and various degrees of fracture-dislocation occur which may be unstable.

A particular type of hyperextension injury is becoming increasingly common in elderly people who have degenerative changes in the cervical spine (cervical spondylosis). During the temporary deformity at the moment of hyperextension, the cord is severely bruised between the thickened protruding hardened disc anteriorly and the neural arches and ligamenta flava posteriorly (Figs. 1.20 and 1.21). There is often minor bony damage which is not visible on X-rays. The lesion is *stable*.

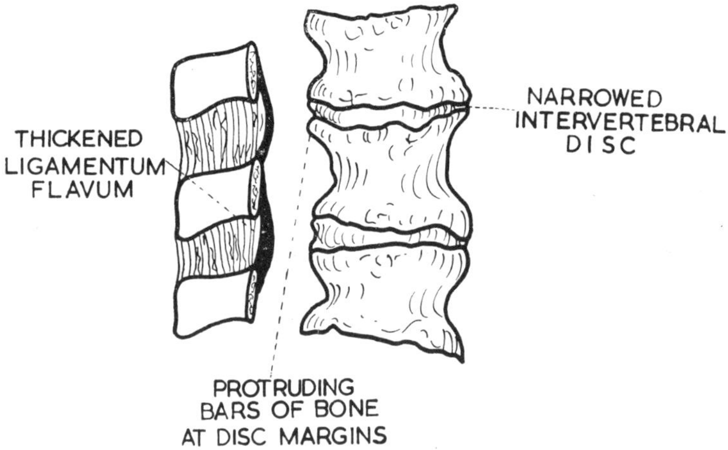

Fig. 1.20 Bone deformities associated with cervical spondylosis; note the protuberant posterior aspects of the discs and the bulky ligamenta flava.

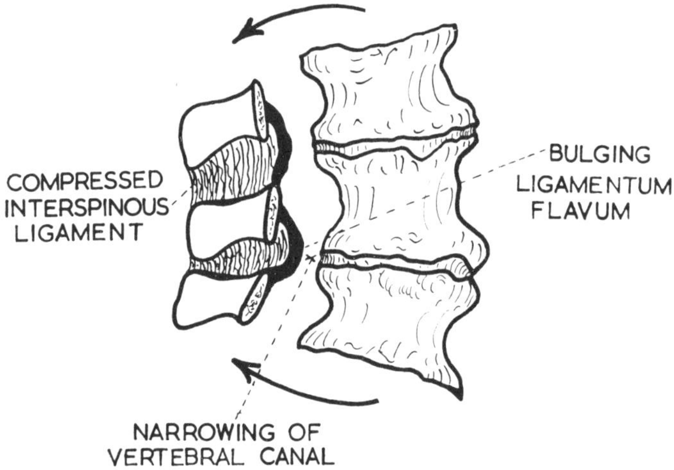

Fig. 1.21 The results of hyperextension—at the point marked X, the spinal cord can be crushed between protuberant disc anteriorly and bulging ligamentumflavum posteriorly.

5. *Lateral flexion*

Severe lateral flexion may injure the *cervical* or *lumbar* regions. Lateral wedge fracture can occur at both levels and unstable fracture-dislocation is likely in cervical examples. Pure lateral flexion is uncommon.

6. *Direct injury*

Some spinal injuries are produced by the violence of a direct blow. This arises, for example, when a person is struck by a falling or flying object of any size, or when a moving person strikes some solid object in the region of his spine.

Examples. (a) A blow on the back by falling masonry or building material or fragments of debris from an explosion; (b) A motor cyclist thrown from his motor cycle and striking a wall or part of the road or kerb; (c) A gun-shot wound.

Result. One or more parts of the vertebra are shattered and sometimes sheared (Fig. 1.22).

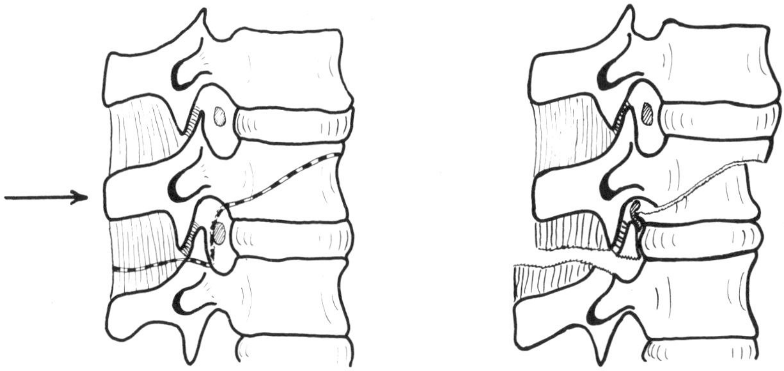

Fig. 1.22 A shear fracture. The arrow indicates the site of a direct force of sufficient magnitude to displace one vertebra horizontally on the one beneath. The important distinction is that the whole vertebra has slid at the fracture site. The dotted line indicates the line of the fracture and associated ligament damage. The cord is likely to be compressed.

7. *Violent muscle contraction*

When the body is subjected to any violent stress, the muscles react to protect all parts from gross deformity. Frequently the combined effects of muscular contraction and deformity result in fractures at the sites of bony attachment of these muscles. Commonly, transverse and spinous processes are fractured in this way.

All combinations of these forces can occur and their effects are modified by the speed with which they are applied—new types of spinal injuries are being seen, the results of high velocity road traffic accidents.

Spinal cord damage *can* occur in all these examples, whether stable or unstable.

Pathological fractures are seen in the spine as in any other part of the skeleton. A common example of conditions weakening the bone is osteoporosis in elderly people, in whom wedge fractures of the thoracic vertebrae can occur due to minor falls. Both primary and secondary tumours can cause weakening of the vertebrae and in these, spinal cord compression is common.

Intervertebral disc lesions

Any of the causes mentioned above can result in damage to the intervertebral disc; if the annulus tears, central soft disc material can squirt (prolapse) through the breach into the spinal canal and compress the spinal cord itself or it may only impact in the intervertebral canal and squeeze one of the segmental nerves. *Cord pressure* from a prolapsed intervertebral disc is a serious emergency (Fig. 1.23).

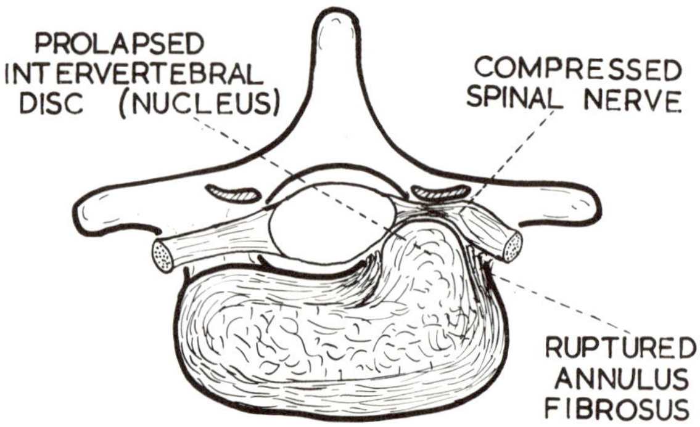

Fig. 1.23 Rupture of part of the annulus fibrosus and prolapse of nucleus pulposus material which has compressed the nerve roots; a more medially placed prolapse could compress the spinal cord itself.

Acute disc lesions with prolapse may follow an accident but some examples are apparently spontaneous or follow minor strains. A further consideration of disc derangements is given on page 45.

2. The Management of Vertebral Fractures

First aid and transport

In vertebral injuries, first-aid measures to prevent damage to the cord rank in importance with moving the patient to safety, controlling haemorrhage and maintaining respiration.

Any injured patient complaining of back or neck pain, abnormal sensation in the limbs or trunk, numbness or loss of movement anywhere, should be treated as having possible spinal damage. Such damage should be considered *unstable*.

Vertebral fractures or dislocations may be associated with damage to the spinal cord at the moment of injury. Alternatively, and even more tragically, the cord may be injured subsequent to a simple vertebral injury because the patient has not been treated with due care.

Many of the techniques used in the management of uncomplicated vertebral fractures and dislocations are also used in the management of cases in which the spinal cord has been injured. The choice of the method of treatment will be decided after consideration of *all* the medical and nursing requirements. In this chapter the methods used in the treatment of the injured vertebral column will be considered; the additional measures necessary if the spinal cord is involved are dealt with later. *Some of the treatments employing the use of plaster jackets or beds or braces as described for vertebral fractures will not be used if there is also a spinal cord injury*. The reasons will be explained on subsequent pages.

The spine itself must not be flexed, extended nor twisted in any way during transport. Poor lifting, which could result in such deformity, is demonstrated in Figure 2.1.

Sufficient help is essential to enable the patient to be lifted 'in one piece.' In one method sufficient hands are insinuated under the patient in the position in which he lies so that this alignment is preserved while he is lifted on to a firm stretcher arranged with pillows or blankets which support the natural curves of the body. A better method, necessitating fewer hands but requiring just as much care, is to roll the patient as shown in Figures 2.2 to 2.8. It can be performed by two people if the neck is uninjured, but three people are desirable in cervical injuries.

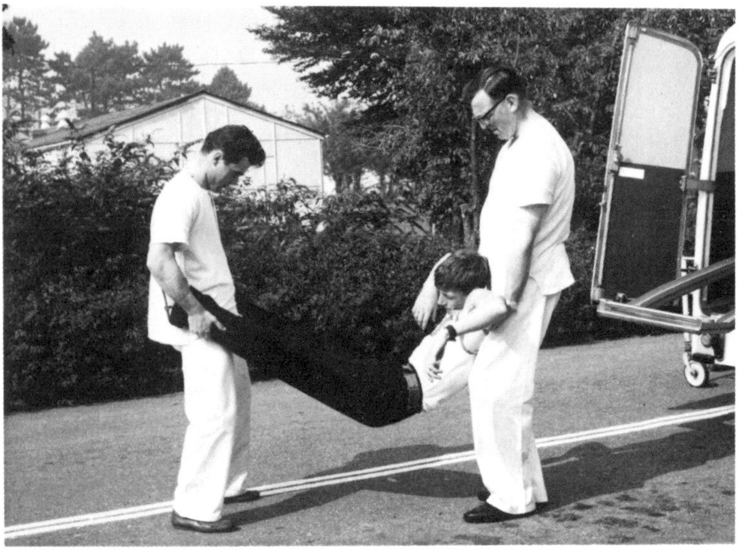

Fig. 2.1 Bad lifting likely to inflict serious damage to the spinal cord if there is an unstable fracture or dislocation.

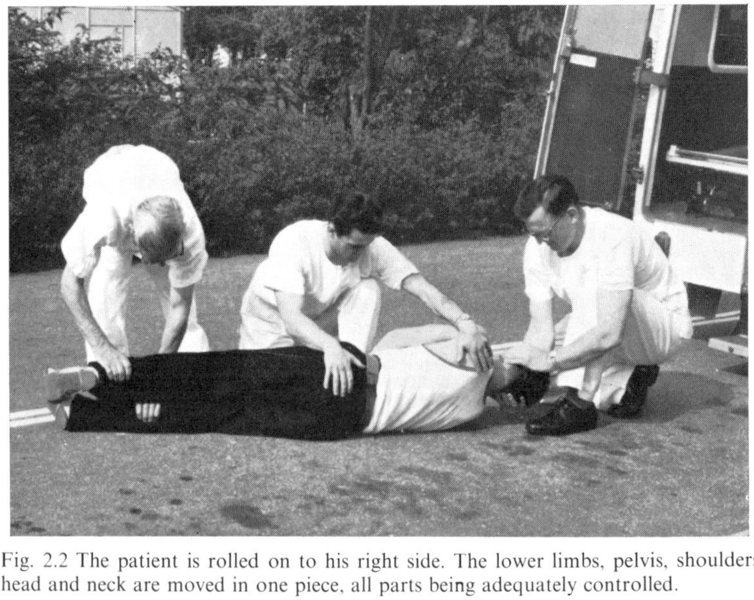

Fig. 2.2 The patient is rolled on to his right side. The lower limbs, pelvis, shoulders, head and neck are moved in one piece, all parts being adequately controlled.

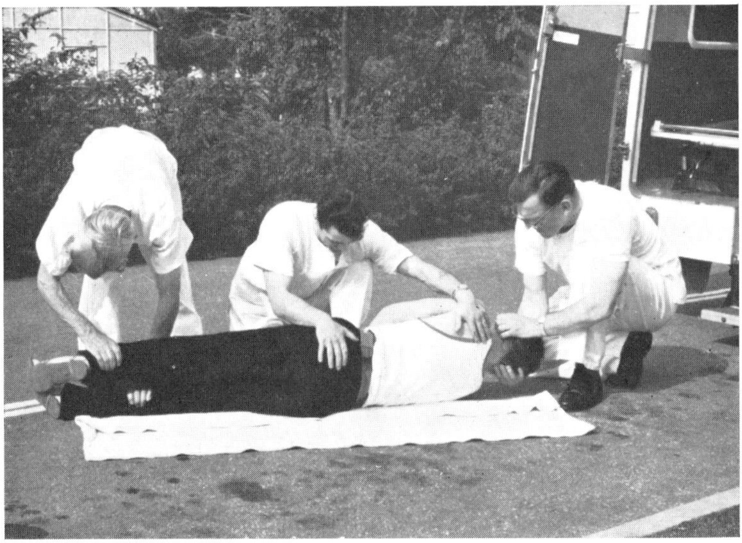

Fig. 2.3 A stretcher canvas, folded lengthwise, is placed alongside the patient.

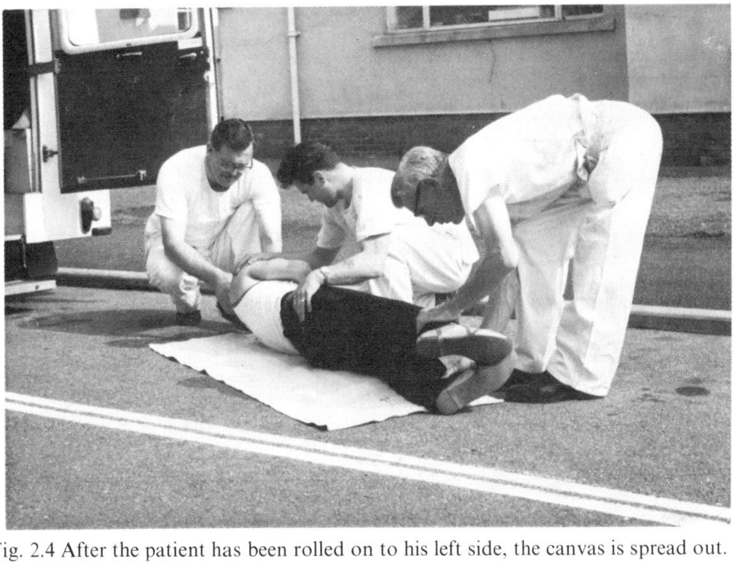

Fig. 2.4 After the patient has been rolled on to his left side, the canvas is spread out.

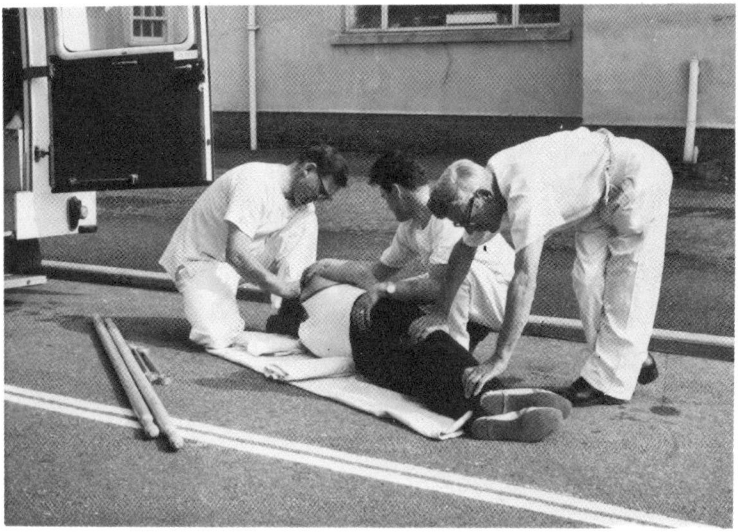

Fig. 2.5 A rolled towel to support the lumbar curve and a firm pad or a sandbag for the head are placed in position. The pad for the head supports the neck in a neutral position, neither extended nor flexed.

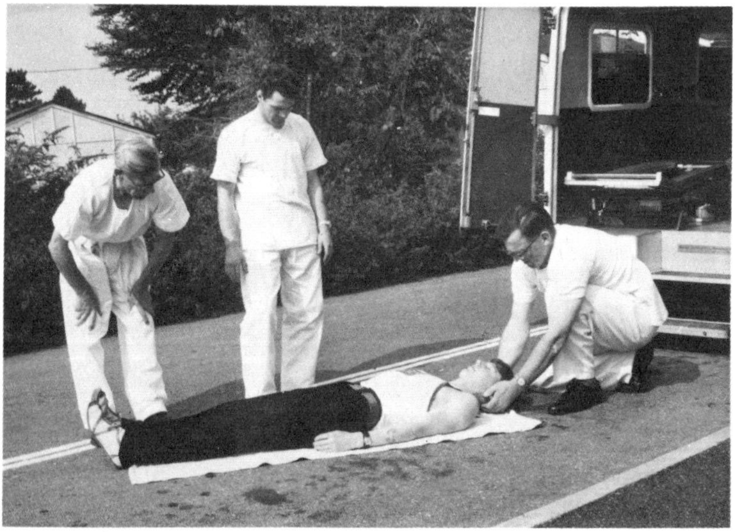

Fig. 2.6 The patient is rolled on to his back, the head remaining supported throughout.

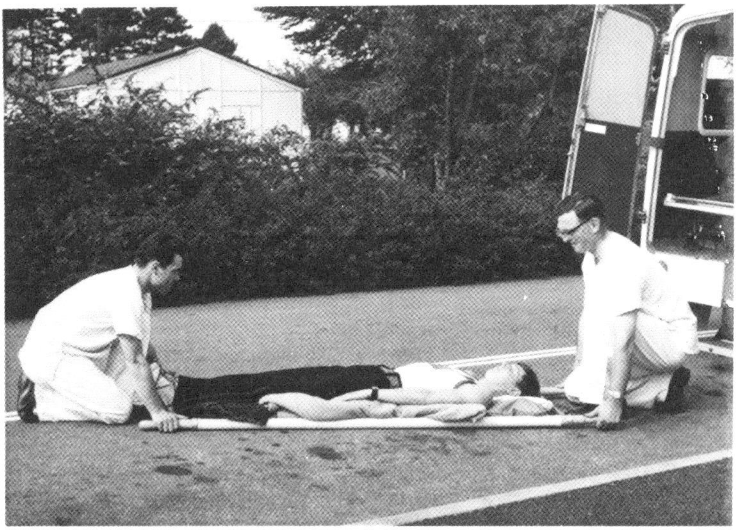

Fig. 2.7 Sandbags are placed on either side of the head to control rotation at the neck. Poles are inserted and the metal spacers applied.

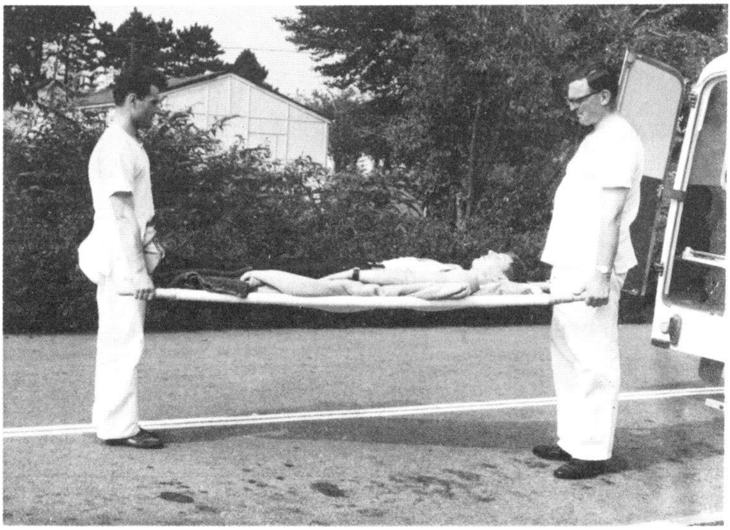

Fig. 2.8 The patient is lifted gently and kept horizontal.

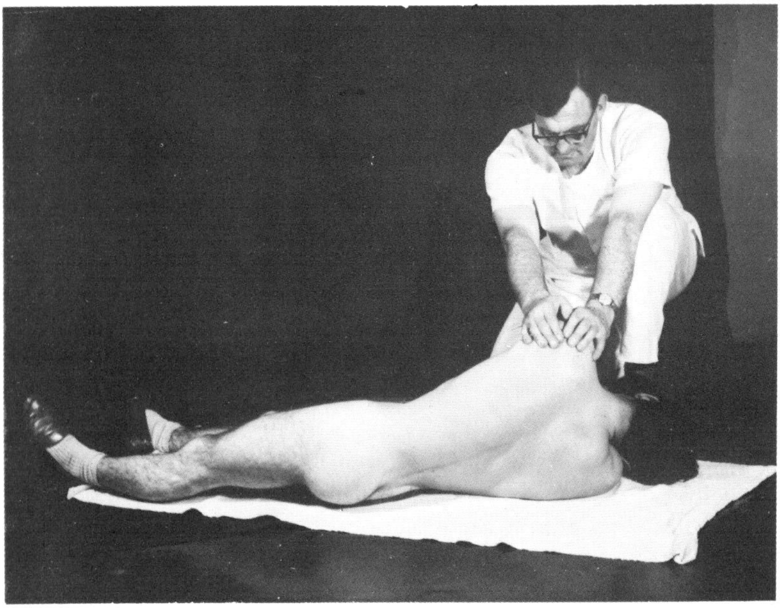

Fig. 2.9 Rolling can be dangerous, especially in the presence of a flexion-rotation injury to the thoraco-lumbar region. In this case, the shoulders are rolled but the pelvis has been left behind.

The important thing is that the natural alignment of the spine is not distorted during transfer on to the stretcher; rolling, unless in one piece, can be just as dangerous as flexion (Fig. 2.9).

The use of the canvas, poles and spacers facilitates further lifting on and off standard ambulance stretchers and X-ray tables. Before transport, remove any hard or sharp objects from the patient's pockets.

Respiratory difficulties may occur. The airway must be kept clear and if assisted breathing is required, positive pressure respiration is best since it involves less violent activity; either mouth-to-mouth breathing or an insufflator should be used. (Any blood or vomitus must be removed before positive pressure respiration is employed.) The prone position is distressing for patients with impaired respiration and is indicated only when there is bleeding from the mouth, or if unconsciousness prevails with the possibility of vomiting.

Hospital management

On arrival at hospital the patient is not disturbed until examined by a doctor and X-rayed. Depending on the findings and, perhaps, special investigations such as lumbar puncture and myelography, treatment will be directed.

Choice of treatment will be dictated by:

1. The presence or absence of cord damage
2. The degree of displacement at the site of injury
3. Whether or not the injury is *stable*
4. Whether or not there is an open wound
5. Associated injuries.

It is not proposed to give in detail the treatment required for each type of fracture; this constitutes a medical consideration. Different methods of treatment which may be ordered are listed below.

1. *Nursing free in bed*

This is satisfactory for stable fractures such as wedged lumbar or thoracic vertebrae, isolated fractures of transverse or spinous processes. The patient is allowed to lie in whatever position is most comfortable and encouraged to increase his mobility as local pain settles. On medical instruction, exercises to strengthen the extensor muscles are performed and, as soon as pain free, the patient may be allowed up. Exercises should become increasingly vigorous until as full movement as possible is re-attained (Fig. 2.10).

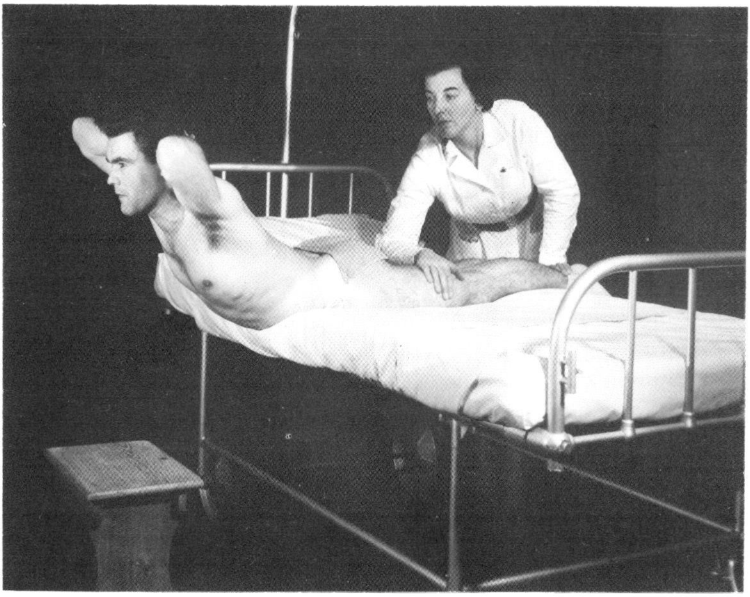

Fig. 2.10 Vigorous back extension exercises.

2. *Nursing free in bed with a sorbo rubber, plaster or polythene collar*

This is convenient for stable fractures of the neck (Figs. 2.11 to 2.13). A collar acts by restricting movement; it is not a means of complete fixation.

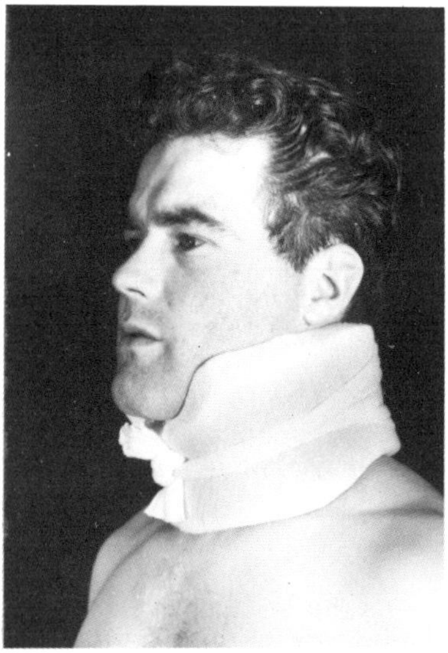

Fig. 2.11 Home-made collar consisting of a strip of one inch sorbo rubber enclosed in a sleeve of stockinette; a cup can be fashioned to accommodate the chin.

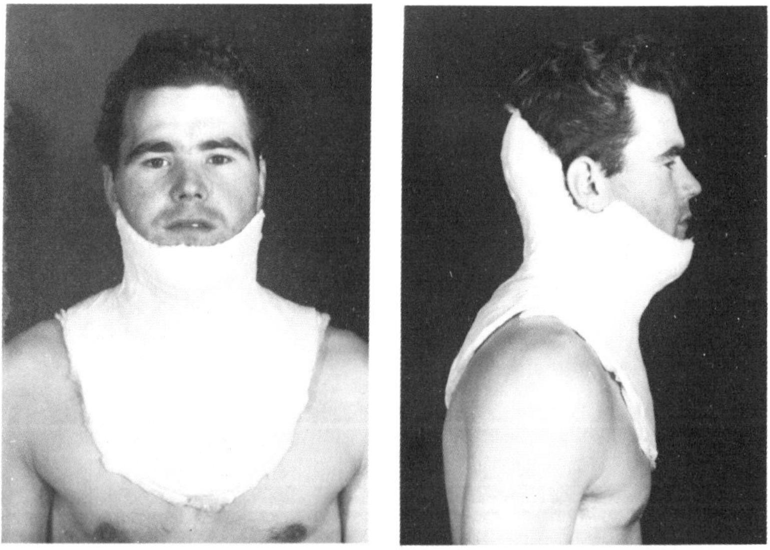

Fig. 2.12 A plaster of Paris 'Doll's' collar. It is comfortable if well made.

3. *Plaster of Paris fixation*

Fractures of the thoracic or lumbar spine *without paraplegia* may be protected in a plaster jacket extending from the pubis to the manubrium (Fig. 2.14). This used to be applied in a position of hyperextension

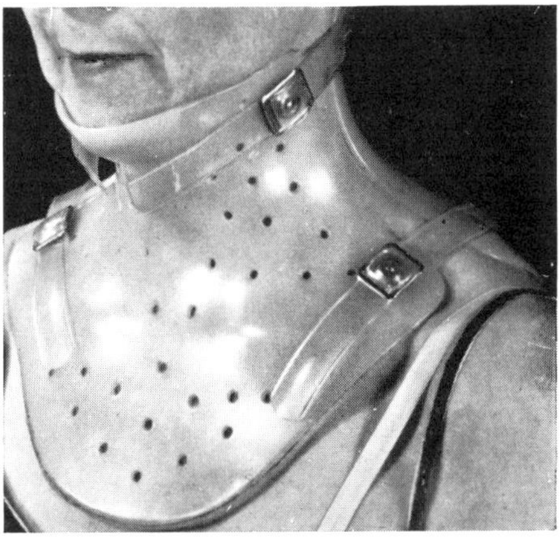

Fig. 2.13 A polythene collar. It can be washed and must be made to measure from a plaster mould.

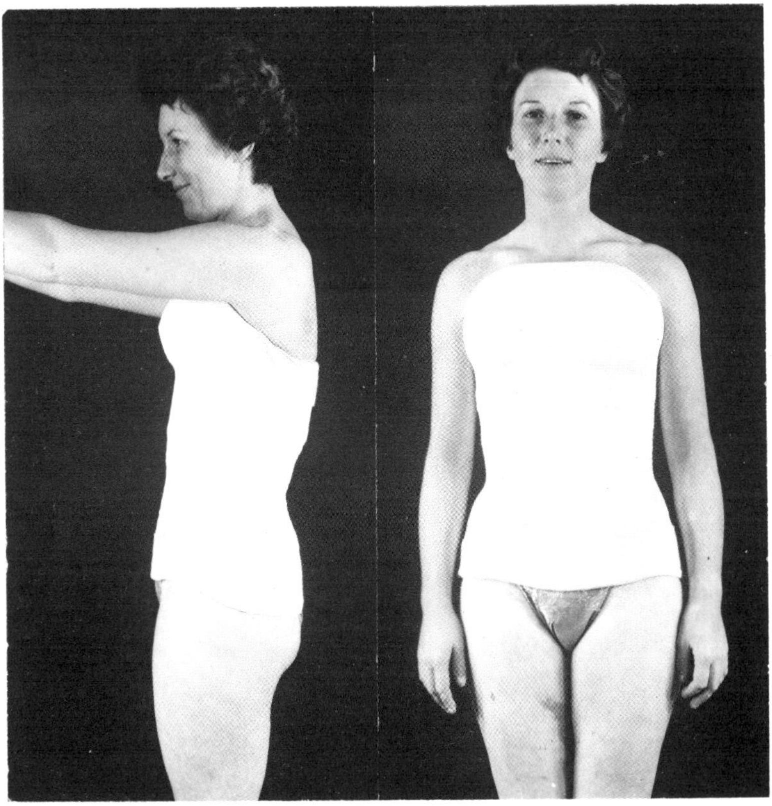

Fig. 2.14 Plaster jacket. It reaches from the pubes to the manubrium.

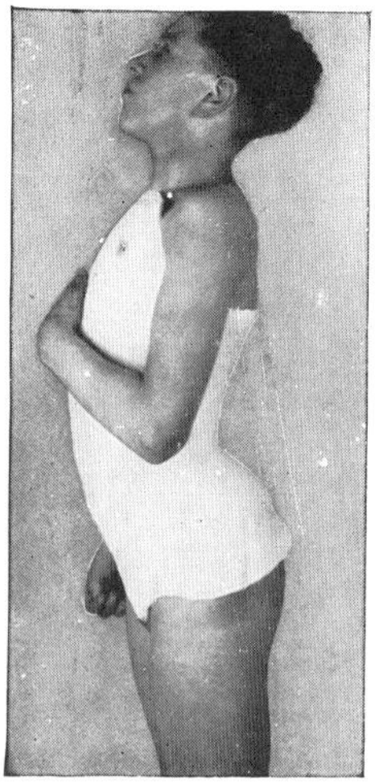

Fig. 2.15 Plaster jacket in hyperextension.

(Fig. 2.15) but it is now considered quite appropriate to apply a plaster jacket with the patient standing or sitting in a normal anatomical postion and, if necessary, after a period of bed rest. However, in the presence of a painful fracture, this may be impossible and in these

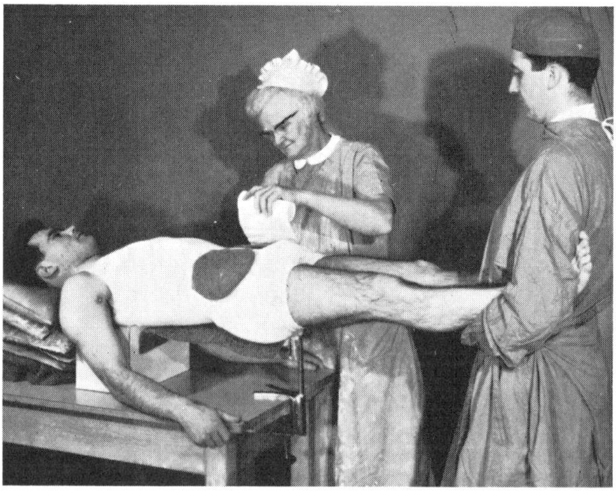

Fig. 2.16 Application of a plaster jacket. The patient lies with his sacrum supported on a steel prop and with his shoulders on a box. His legs are supported by an assistant and, if conscious, he steadies himself by gripping the sides of the table. Pieces of felt protect the iliac spines, sacrum and spinous processes of the vertebral column. When ordered, some hyperextension can be achieved by lowering the legs. As is the case with all body casts, the plaster must be applied firmly and moulded carefully; on standing, unless this instruction has been observed, the cast becomes very loose.

circumstances a plaster may be applied with the patient supine and supported on a prop (Fig. 2.16).

Neck fractures may have to be immobilised in a Minerva plaster (Fig. 2.17) and during its application the head may be held flexed, neutral or extended, depending on the type of fracture. As is the case with plaster jackets, the Minerva plaster may be applied with the patient

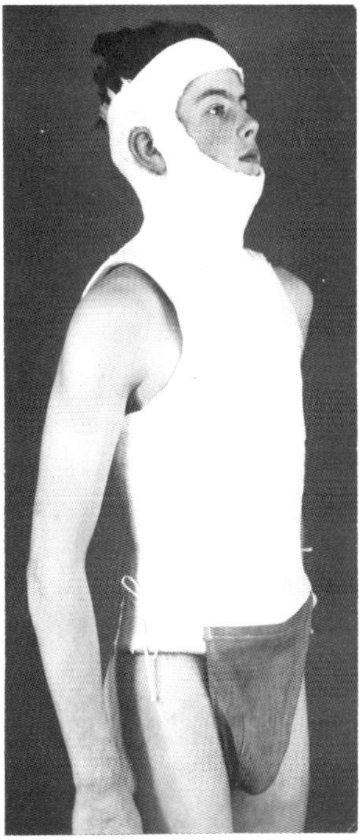

Fig. 2.17 Minerva plaster. It affords good fixation of the whole cervical spine.

supine, using a support as shown in Figure 2.18. The length of time for such plaster fixation is very variable, but for an unstable cervical fracture or dislocation, three or four months is a common period.

Following removal of the plaster, a less rigid fixation may be advised, using a collar, as described above, for the neck, or some type of spinal support for the trunk (Figs. 2.19 and 2.20). Mobilisation exercises may be prescribed.

It should be noted that sometimes plaster immobilisation is preceded by reduction of a fracture or dislocation. Frequently, however, such a procedure is not required and the plaster cast is applied only to protect the part from further displacement. During the application of plaster casts, the usual care in lifting and manipulating the patient is employed; these patients are very apprehensive, and an effort should be made to explain step by step what is going to be done so that they can relax with confidence.

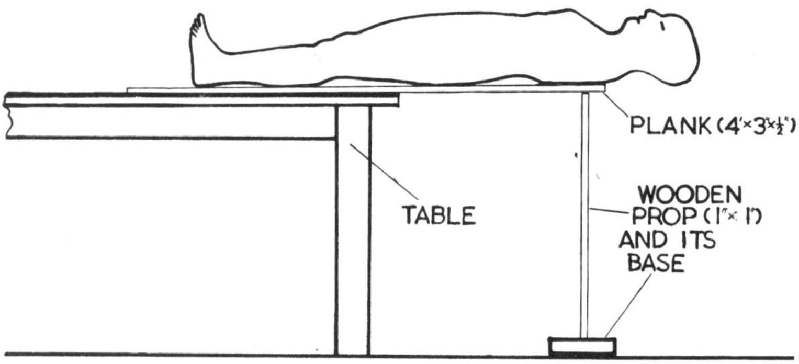

A

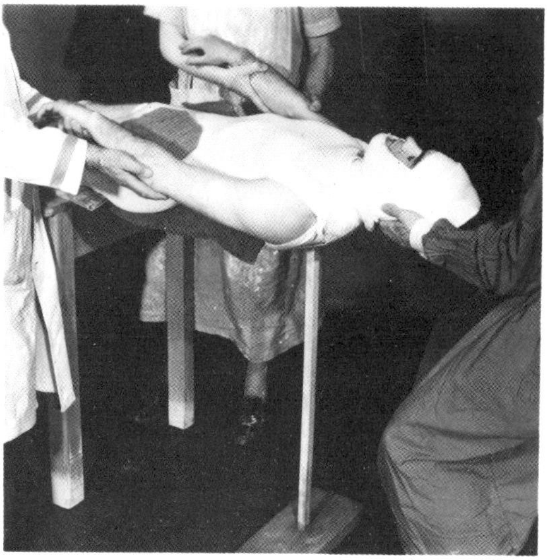

B

Fig. 2.18 Application of a Minerva jacket in supine position. A, Shows patient lying along a thin wooden plank which is supported near its end on a prop. His head is held by the doctor in charge and his arms by assistants on either side. Another assistant steadies the pelvis.

B, The surgeon sits and has comfortable control of the patient's head. Before laying him on the plank, the latter is overlaid by a piece of felt measuring nine by eighteen inches; he wears a stockinette vest and further felt pads protect the iliac spines. Wool rolls encircle both the patient and plank so that at the completion of the plaster, the plank can be slid easily from inside. Plaster rolls and slabs should be applied firmly and the waist line exaggerated for the iliac crests will support much of the cast's weight rather than this being borne by the shoulders. Ear holes are cut after completion.

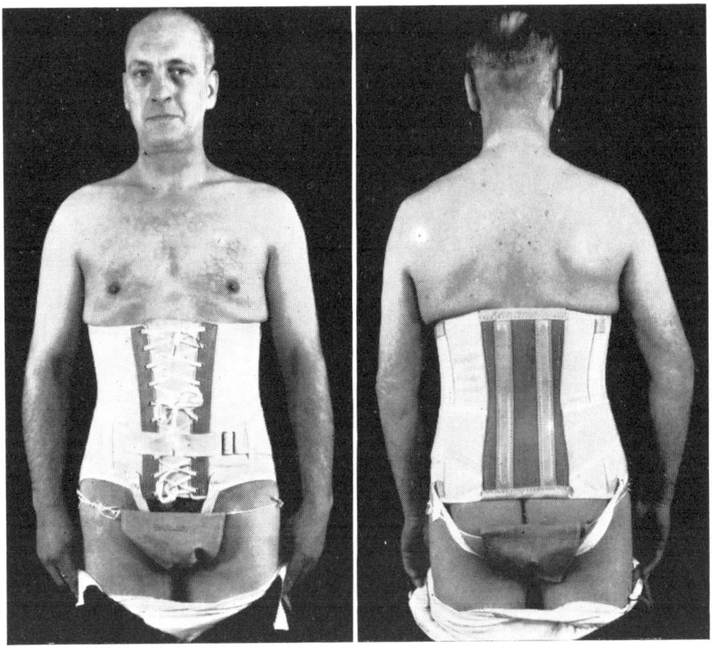

Fig. 2.19 A Goldthwaite spinal support. It is made to measure from a plaster posterior slab.

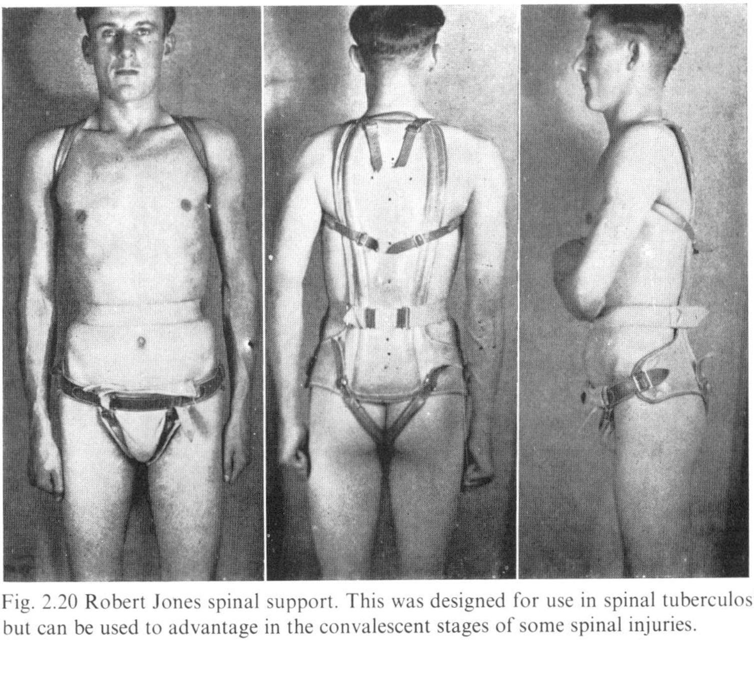

Fig. 2.20 Robert Jones spinal support. This was designed for use in spinal tuberculosis but can be used to advantage in the convalescent stages of some spinal injuries.

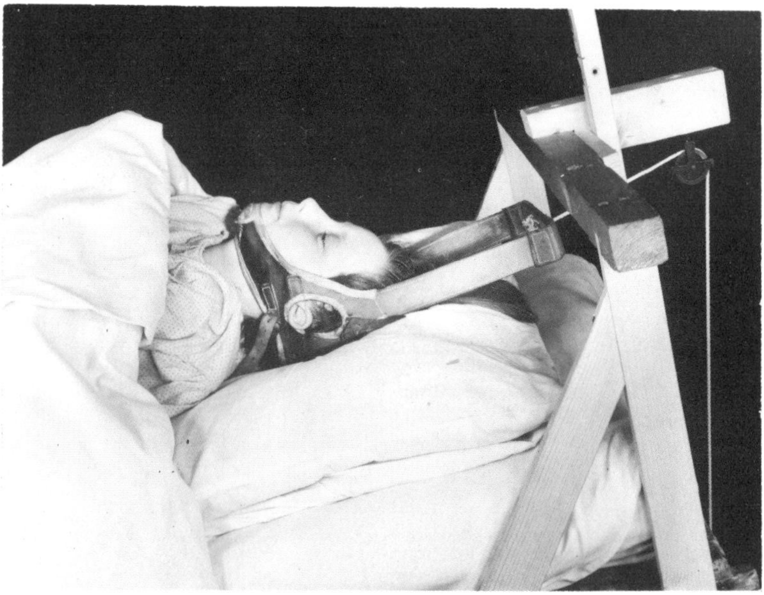

Fig. 2.21 Head traction using a Glisson sling. Note the straps which must be tightened so as to support evenly both chin and occiput.

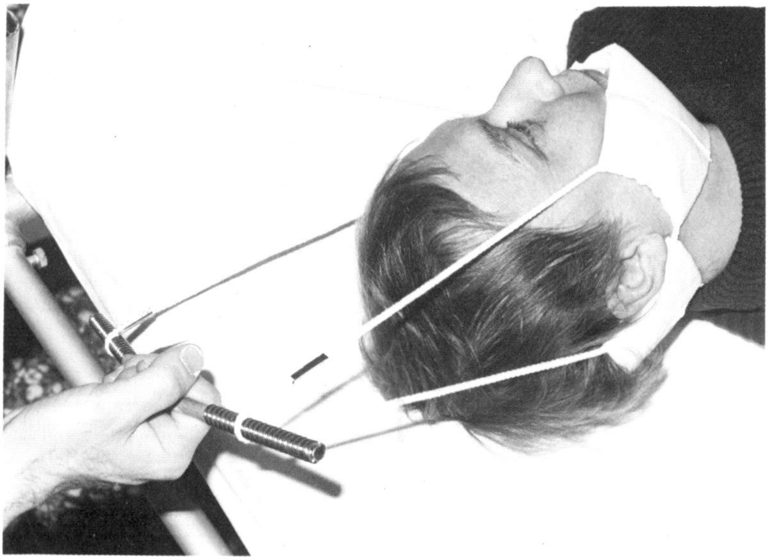

Fig. 2.22 Head traction using Zimmer sling and spreader bar is very useful for controlling the head and neck during transport and radiography.

4. *Traction in fractures or dislocations of the cervical spine*

Traction may be applied to the head by a harness (halter) under the chin and occiput, or by calipers applied to some part of the cranium.

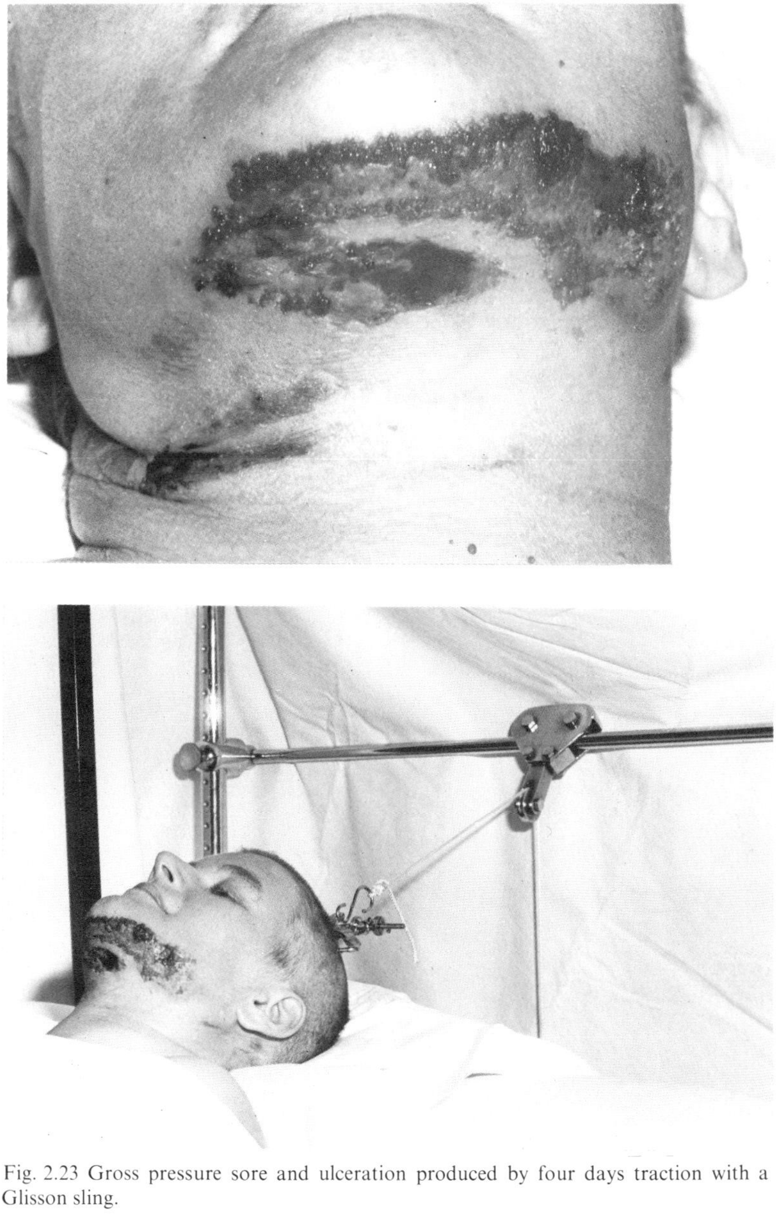

Fig. 2.23 Gross pressure sore and ulceration produced by four days traction with a Glisson sling.

There are several methods and techniques of applying traction and each has its indications and advocates.

Halter traction (Figs. 2.21 and 2.22) is of use as a *temporary measure* only. The head can be controlled during First Aid and in transportation, and also while the patient is undergoing X-ray examination either in bed or on an accident trolley. It should only be used with light weights of 1 to 2 kg (2 to 4 lb) for short periods. With greater weights and over long periods it can be extremely uncomfortable and if applied for more than a few hours there is a very real danger of the skin beneath the chin and below the occiput becoming sore and even ulcerated (Fig. 2.23).

With *skull traction* much greater forces can be employed: 2 to 4 kg (5 to 10 lb) is common and even 10 to 20 kg (25 to 50 lb) can be used for special purposes. The head of the bed or turning frame needs to be elevated to prevent the tendency for the patient to be dragged little by little towards the head end.

There are several types of skull calipers of which the common examples are:

1. *Crutchfield calipers* (Figs. 2.24 to 2.27). These calipers can be inserted into the dome of the skull under local anaesthesia. The points are located into holes drilled into the outer table of the skull. The inner table is not penetrated.

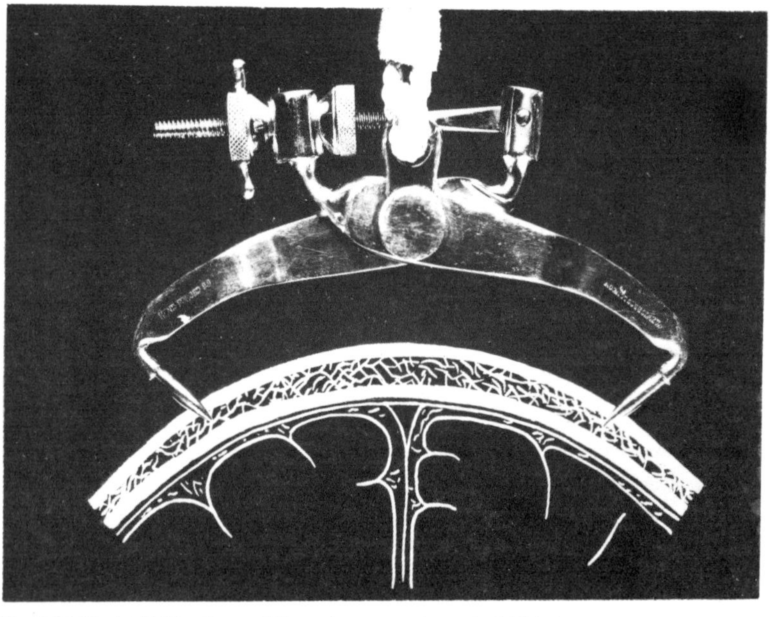

Fig. 2.24 Crutchfield calipers. The points pass through drill holes in the outer table of the skull only.

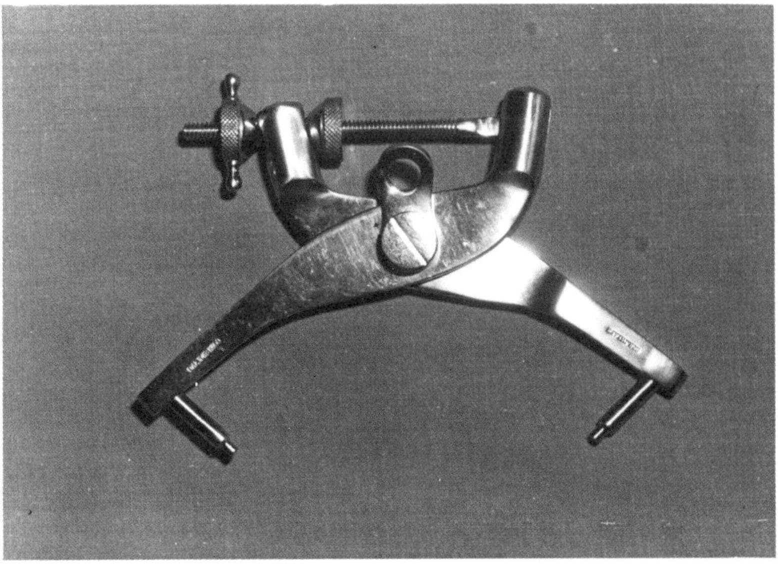

Fig. 2.25 Modern Crutchfield calipers with truncated points which avoid the possibility of penetrating the inner table of the skull vault.

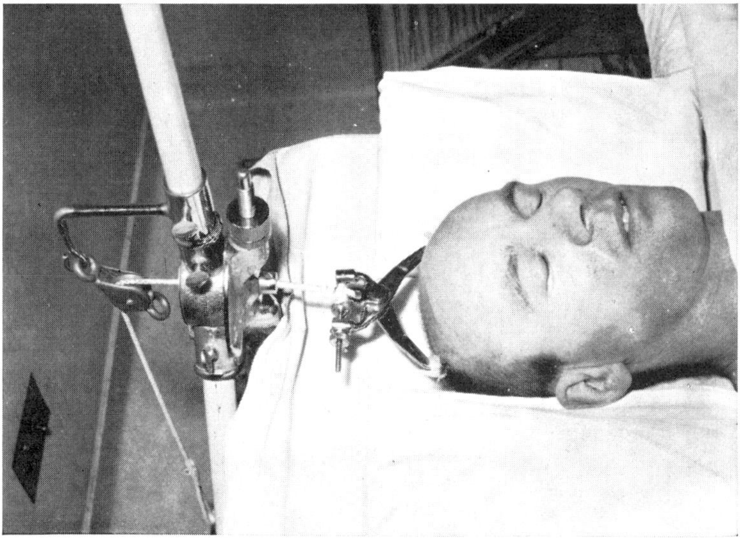

Fig. 2.26 Head traction using Crutchfield calipers and a Stryker frame.

2. *Blackburn calipers.* These are heavier and more substantial than the Crutchfield design and require skin incisions and drill holes in the skull above and behind the level of the ears (Figs. 2.28 and 2.29).

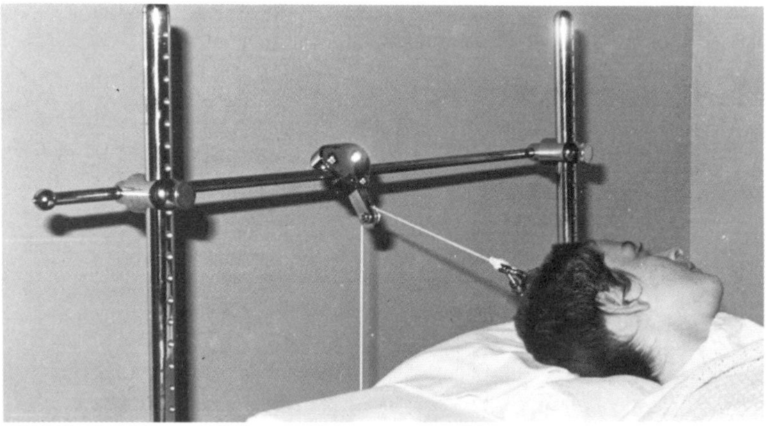

A

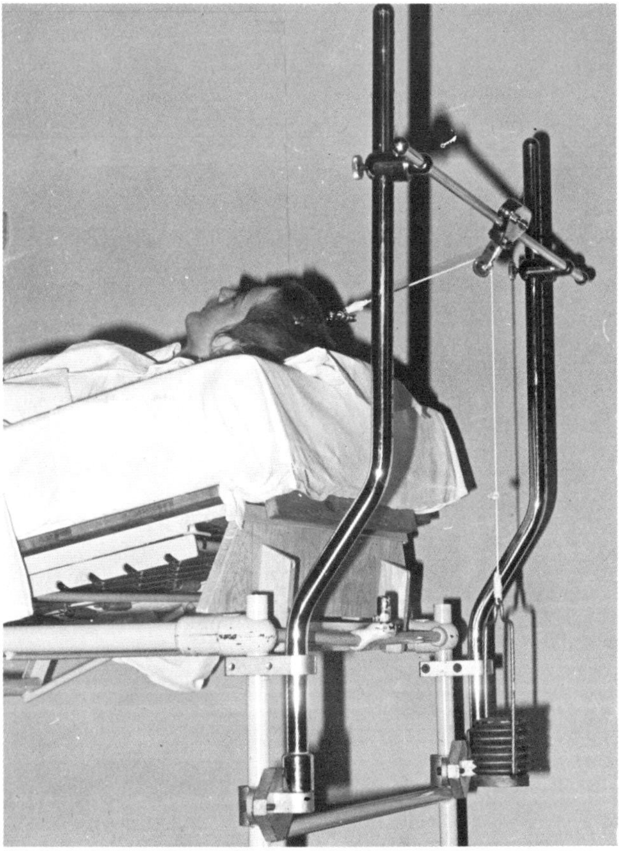

B

Fig. 2.27 A, Head traction using Crutchfield calipers. B, A skeletal traction unit attached to a Fowler bed, with a slight elevation of the head end.

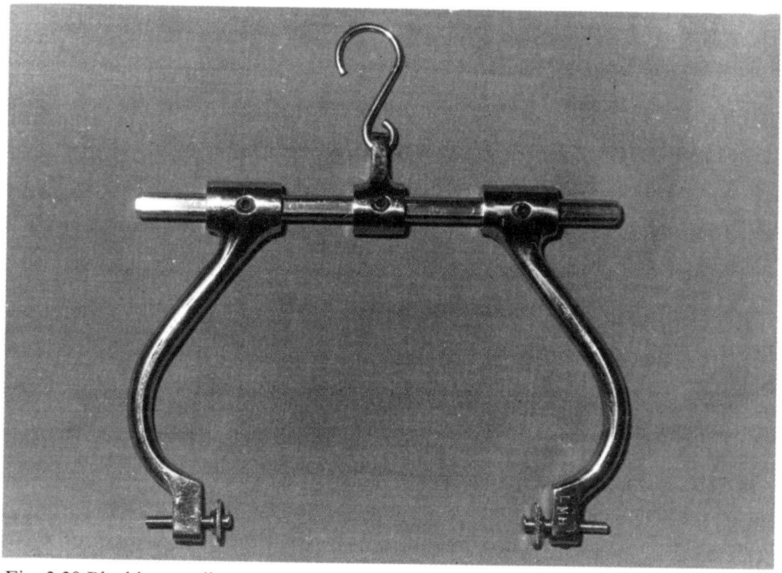

Fig. 2.28 Blackburn calipers.

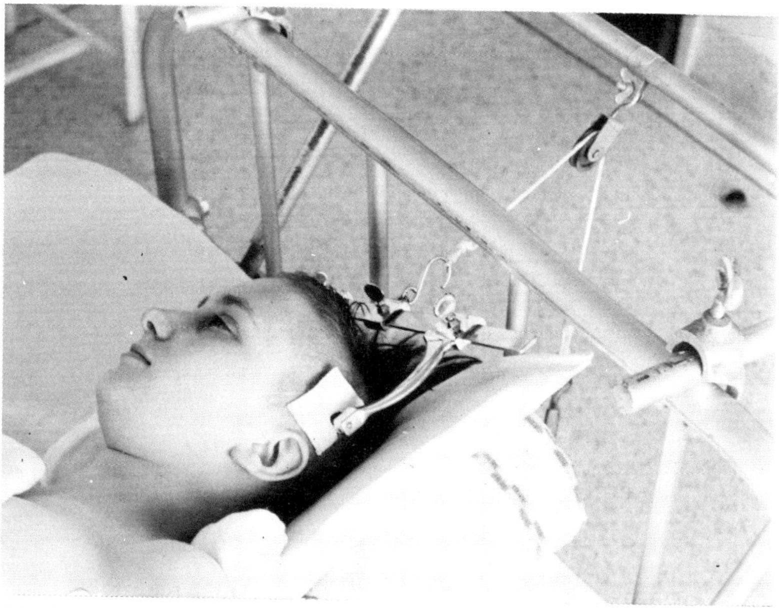

Fig. 2.29 Head traction using Blackburn calipers.

particularly when in an ordinary bed; this does not apply so much when a Stryker turning frame is used.

The transverse bar which holds together the two side pieces of the apparatus tends to make the turning of the patient more difficult,

3. *Cone calipers* (Fig. 2.30). These are similar to the Blackburn

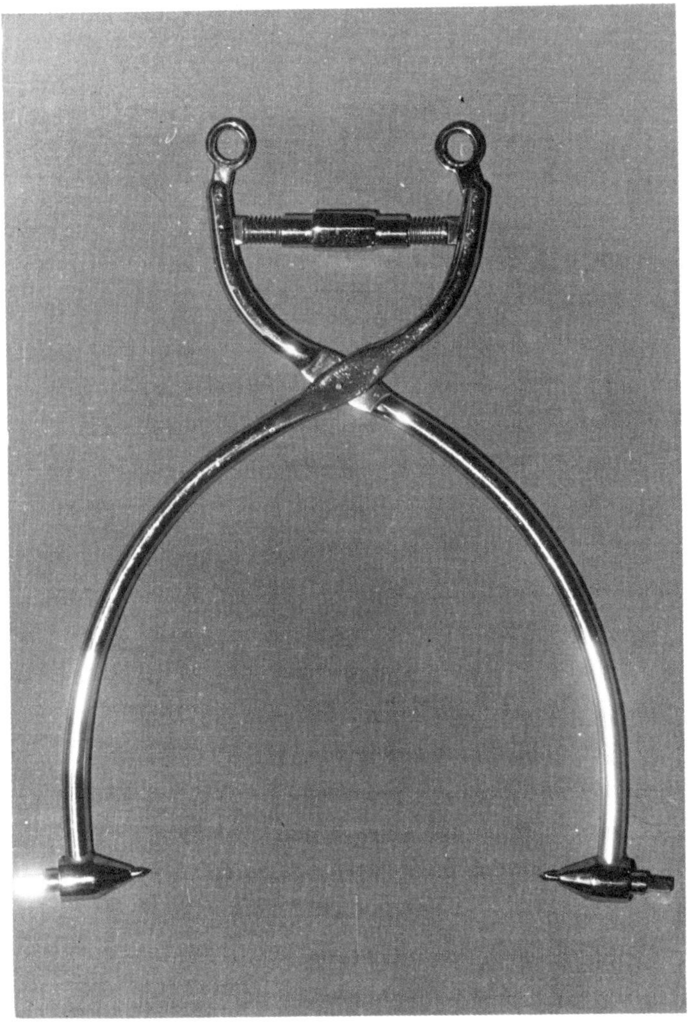

Fig. 2.30 Cone calipers.

pattern and are inserted into the lateral aspects of the skull with the aid of small drills which have a pre-set depth, being designed so as not to penetrate the skull. The advantage of this piece of apparatus is that it is lighter and easier to apply than the Blackburn caliper.

4. *Vinke caliper* (Fig. 2.31). These skull tongs are less well known but nevertheless a very useful lightweight caliper, again requiring

special drill holes and an undercutting tool for its insertion. It has the special advantage of fitting snugly to the sides of the head.

The regular inspection of any of these calipers is the duty of both doctor and nurse. It is important to see that locking nuts are secure and that the small incisions or drill holes are kept scrupulously clean. The scalp should have been shaved locally and these small wounds carefully dressed. If they become infected there is a serious possibility of local osteomyelitis or even extradural abscess.

Special care is required in the case of children, and it should be noted that Crutchfield calipers can rarely be used because of the small diploic space and soft bone.

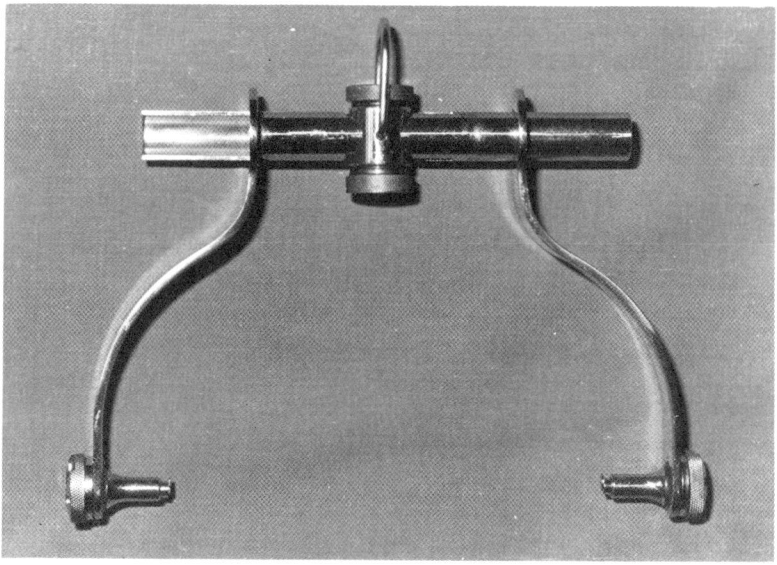

Fig. 2.31 Vinke calipers.

Traction may be used both for the purpose of obtaining reduction of a fracture or dislocation, and the maintenance of the reduced position in subsequent weeks. In the reduction of dislocations, bursting fractures or fracture dislocations, heavy traction may be all that is necessary. In some instances reduction by traction may be assisted by general anaesthesia and muscle relaxants. X-rays are taken at regular intervals until reduction is achieved and then the amount of weight required to maintain the reduction and alignment is adjusted according to the weight of the patient. Very occasionally a Minerva plaster may be applied incorporating the skull calipers but this technique is used far less commonly now than in the past.

The fracture or fracture dislocation should be maintained in the reduced position until satisfactory healing has occurred.

Patients on skull traction require special attention during nursing procedures. The traction is never released and when a patient is turned or moved the cord weights should be controlled by a senior person. The traction cord should not be fouled by the head of the bed or frame, and the patient's head can be supported on a small pillow or latex foam cushion; care should be taken to see that hair is not allowed to bunch up or get entangled; indeed, it is an advantage to have the head shaved or the hair cut short when a period of prolonged traction is anticipated.

It should be noted that skull traction is often used as a therapeutic measure in cases other than those presenting with injury: e.g. cervical spondylosis or destructive disease of the cervical vertebrae.

5. *Operations*

Manipulation under anaesthetic. This technique is sometimes employed in reducing dislocations, most commonly of the cervical spine. It is an expert manoeuvre requiring great care for, once anaesthetised,

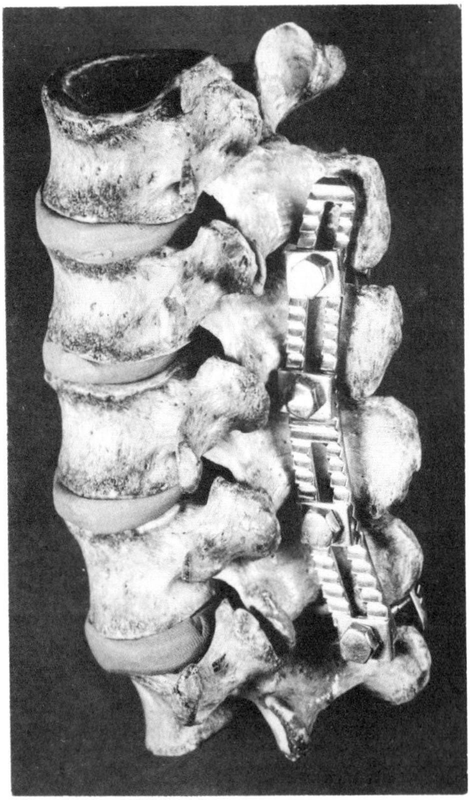

Fig. 2.32 Lumbar spine with Meurig-Williams plates applied.

the patient no longer possesses his own protective reflexes to prevent further gross displacement and possible cord damage. After reduction has been achieved, fixation by plaster or traction methods, described above, may be employed.

Open reduction. If closed methods of reduction fail or are contra-indicated, open operation may be necessary. The bones are exposed and the displacement reduced under direct vision.

Internal fixation. Internal fixation is sometimes required after an open reduction or in some unstable but spontaneously reduced fractures or dislocations. It can be achieved by the insertion of various types of plates or rods fastened to the spinous processes or laminae. In the cervical spine the spinous processes may be tethered together by stainless steel wire and bone grafts may be used when required. The thoracolumbar spine has large spinous processes which are suitable for plating (Fig. 2.32) but wiring is more usual in the cervical

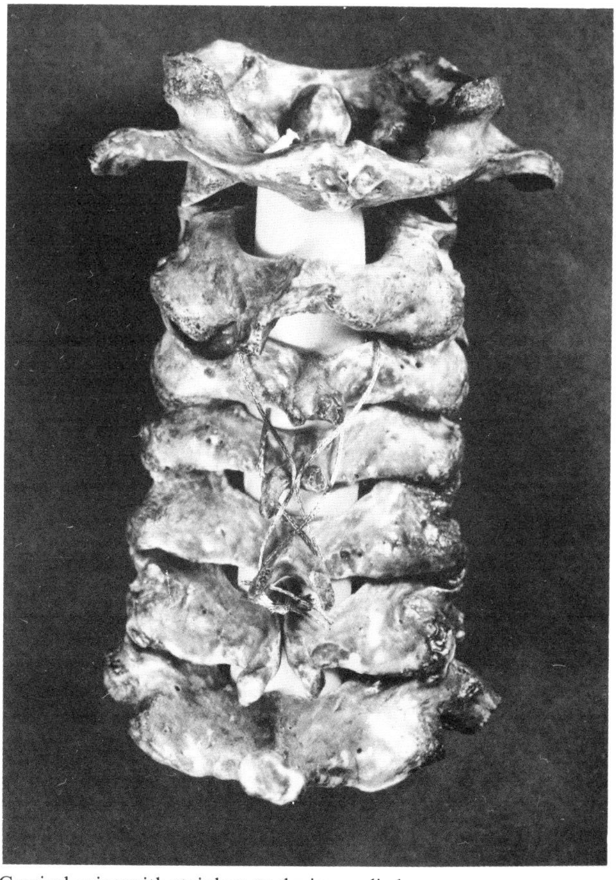

Fig. 2.33 Cervical spine with stainless steel wire applied.

region (Fig. 2.33). *Internal fixation is not to be regarded as a substitute for good nursing.* Expertise and care to maintain a normal anatomical alignment of head and shoulders are required at all times.

Spinal fusion. Stability and relief of symptoms can occur only after healing of the injured part. In some instances, experience tells that healing is likely to be unsound or protracted; instability and pain can result. In such cases, arthrodesis of the injured vertebrae may be performed, so that, once united, no displacement can occur. This may be done early and be combined with wiring in the cervical region, or plating in the thoraco-lumbar region. In other cases it is performed as a late procedure because of progressive displacement following what was thought to be an adequate period of immobilisation. Sometimes spinal fusion is performed for persistent pain at the site of injury. It is usually done from the posterior aspect so that laminae, spines and posterior joints become joined in a sheet of solid bone. In another method, the vertebral bodies are arthrodeses by an anterior approach in both the neck and trunk.

Spinal fusions in the lumbar and thoracic regions of patients *without spinal cord injury* usually require a period of immobilisation on a plaster bed and later in a plaster or polythene jacket. In these cases the plaster bed is made before the operation (Figs. 2.34, 2.35, 2.36) but sometimes it is applied with the patient still prone on the operating table. Cervical fusions may be put straight into a Minerva plaster but may be more simply held by a skull traction apparatus. Several vertebrae can be arthrodesed without serious loss of movement except at the atlanto-axial level, where shaking of the head

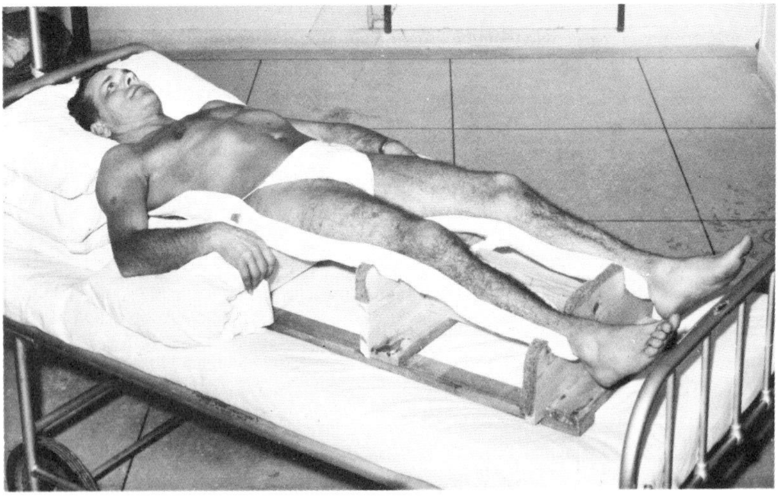

Fig. 2.34 Patient lying in a plaster bed. His arms are supported on pillows. An important adjunct (not shown) is a swivel mirror over the bed head so that a horizontal view of the ward surroundings is available.

occurs, and at the atlanto occipital level where the greater part of nodding takes place. Occasionally fusion is necessary even at these sites.

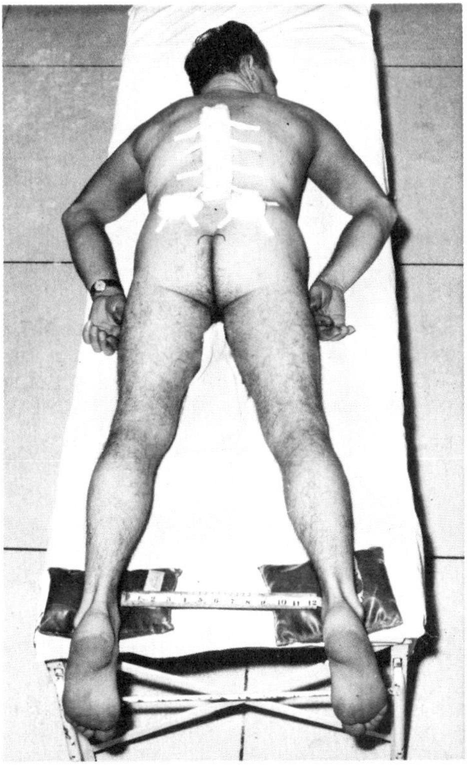

Fig. 2.35 Making a plaster bed. The patient lies prone on a firm surface. His legs are abducted slightly so that the internal malleoli are not more than 13 inches apart, and a sandbag is placed under each ankle so as to flex the knees about five degrees. Care is taken that he lies symmetrically.

The indelible pencil mark at the top of the natal cleft indicates where the plaster is to be cut away in order that a bed pan can be used. The cut-away part must not be more than three inches across at its widest part or discomfort will be experienced.

All bony prominences are protected in the manner shown by thick white wool pads; later these are removed from the cast so that slight hollows remain and there is in consequence no risk of pressure over these bony parts.

Should a head piece be required, it is necessary to arrange the trunk on pillows so that the neck may flex slightly and hyperextension of the finished head piece is avoided.

Debridement of open wounds. All open wounds must be treated by operation. They are cleaned and any dead tissue and foreign bodies are removed together with any loose bone fragments. After adequate surgical toilet the wound is usually closed. In knife and gunshot

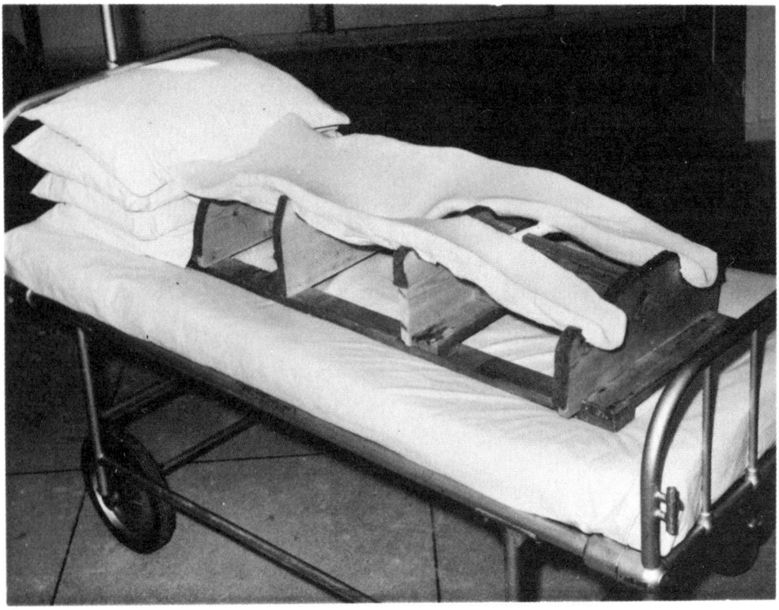

Fig. 2.36 Making a plaster bed. The finished plaster bed is lined with two layers of splint wool covered by stockinette. It is supported on a wooden platform. The minimum height of the plaster is at the buttock, and here it should not be less than four inches. Further, the upright supports in this region must be at least 14 inches apart so as to allow ingress of a bed pan.

wounds, leakage of cerebro-spinalfluid indicates that the meninges have been damaged; this may permit infection to spread to the subarachnoid space and cause meningitis. The use of the modern antibiotics has greatly minimised the risks of this complication occurring.

Laminectomy and exploration of the vertebral canal. This operation is included here although it is only performed when there is evidence of pressure on the spinal cord or nerve roots. In acute injuries the operation may be performed as an emergency; sometimes it is done as a delayed procedure when, for example, some recovery of cord function has occurred but has not continued. To expose the cord, the vertebral canal is opened by removing laminae and spinous processes of several vertebrae (laminectomy). Figure 2.37 shows the extent of laminectomy.

Various structures can press on the cord e.g. bone fragments, a prolapsed portion of an intervertebral disc, or foreign bodies such as shell fragments and bullets in war injuries. In some cases, pressure from excessive callus formation can occur. Occasionally, a nerve leaving the spinal canal is compressed and this can be relieved by unroofing the intervertebral canal through which it makes its exit (foraminotomy).

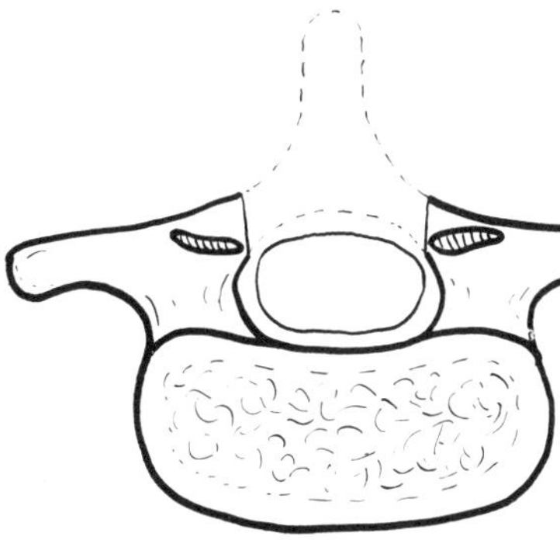

Fig. 2.37 Compare with Fig. 1.2. The extent of bone removal in the operation of laminectomy. If greater access is necessary, parts of the posterior joints can be removed.

Minor injuries to the spinal column

Fractures and dislocations of the spine are usually the result of great violence: the exceptions occur in patients who have a weakness of the vertebrae associated with some bone disease or destructive process. Minor injuries to the spinal column are far more common and arise as a result of smaller forces which produce effects by sprain of the ligaments and muscles which support the vertebral column. The term 'sprain' describes partial rupture of a ligament or muscle and there is frequently severe local pain, as well as radiation down a limb (e.g. sciatica or brachial neuralgia). Everyone is familiar with the severe symptoms that can be produced when a muscle is 'pulled' or an ankle is 'sprained'. In a system as complex as the vertebral column it is not surprising that some of the numerous joints and muscles are injured even in the course of the performance of many day to day activities. Aching backs are indeed a common symptom, and as all spinal movements accompany most activities of daily living it is very difficult to rest the injured parts no matter how small they may be. It is for this reason that many symptoms persist for long periods.

Lesions of an intervertebral disc may follow trauma. The annulus may be sprained or sometimes a complete rupture with prolapse of the nucleus pulposus may occur. The prolapsed material may press on nerves as they escape from the spinal canal or, in the cervical or thoracic regions, press directly on the cord. Acute centrally prolapsed discs in the cervical and thoracic regions constitute surgical emergencies. In the lumbar region, disc prolapses affect the nerves of the cauda equina and often may be treated conservatively. Disc lesions are a common orthopaedic problem, and their management is dealt with more fully in textbooks on orthopaedic nursing; most cases do not follow acutely on an accident.

These minor injuries are the most common examples of trauma to the vertebral column; *they are responsible for much loss of work and disability*. The precipitating cause may have been so minor that it was not noticed and the back or neck pain comes on apparently spontaneously.

Degenerative changes in the spine seen in the elderly or in individuals who have subjected their backs to prolonged repeated stress (e.g. miners) seem to predispose to painful symptoms from such minor injuries; a change of occupation may be advisable.

Pain in the back or neck is a distressing complaint and the nurse should show a kind yet firm sympathy for patients so afflicted; it is never the nurse's duty to label such pains as hysterical or 'functional' and in consequence show impatience or intolerance.

The more severe examples may be admitted to hospital and certain nursing measures may be ordered:

1. *A firmly supported mattress.* A sagging bedspring and mattress allow the trunk to lie in a curve so that with the patient on his back the spine also sags into flexion. Lying on the side deforms the spine into lateral flexion, and lying prone is impossible. Fracture boards underneath the mattress prevent this sagging, but the mattress must not be a thin one as is so frequently seen. It is most punitive to subject someone already in pain to a ridiculously thin 'hard mattress'; it is the underlying support which needs reinforcing.

2. *Traction on the legs* affords considerable relief to many cases of low back pain. Skin traction of 2 kg (5 lb) is applied to each lower limb and the foot of the bed is elevated 6 to 9 cm in to give a counter-pull; details of the technique of application can be found in any orthopaedic nursing textbook.

Sometimes traction is applied to the pelvis by means of a corset, but this is usually found to be less satisfactory and is uncomfortable.

3. *Head traction by a halter* (intermittent) or by skull calipers is sometimes used in painful neck sprains, especially if such an injury has precipitated symptoms associated with cervical osteoarthritis. The direction of the traction is that required for maximum comfort; sometimes the patient is most comfortable with the neck slightly flexed.

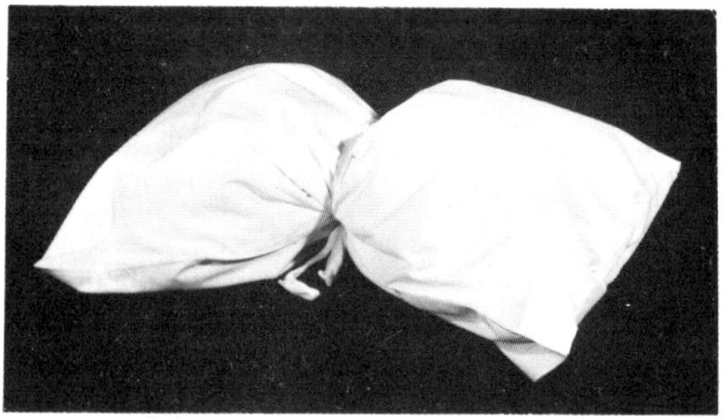

Fig. 2.38 A 'butterfly' pillow.

4. *A butterfly pillow.* Some cases of cervical injury are made comfortable if the neck is slightly hyperextended; this can be achieved by letting the head extend over a pillow tied with tape in the manner shown in Figure 2.38.

5. *Local heat* from a hot water bottle (administered with the usual nursing care and consideration) or hot baths are comforting. (Heat in any form is never applied if the patient has a spinal cord injury.) Other measures include various physiotherapeutic aids and analgesic drugs.

3. The Results of Injury to the Spinal Cord

Injury to the spinal cord is the most serious complication of vertebral trauma. Until the Second World War, it was a common precept that these patients had a hopeless future; they were put into chronic sick hospitals or, more usually, they died. Modern medicine has enabled them to be kept alive and they deserve the highest quality treatment in all respects; only this will enable their further existence to be happy. There is no more catastrophic event than injury to the spinal cord, especially when the site of injury is in the cervical region.

Undoubtedly, nursing of the highest quality is the fundamental requirement, *especially in the vital first few weeks*. The theory of such nursing is quite easy but its practice is difficult, exacting and expensive. Further, not only high orthopaedic standards are necessary but also a working knowledge of other branches of specialised nursing, especially urological and neurosurgical. A free co-operation with physiotherapists, occupational therapists and patient's relatives must be accepted. It is on the hub of the nursing care that all other therapeutic efforts depend, but the nurse must recognise the importance of other experts.

This chapter explains the abnormal physiology which results from a spinal cord injury. After each abnormality has been described, the consequent related principles of management are outlined. Good management is logical and easily understood as a consequence of the disordered physiology. It cannot be overstressed that the secret of successful management lies in *prevention of complications*; once complications occur (and they can occur so very easily even in the best of circumstances) they are very difficult to rectify. Furthermore, one complication leads rapidly to another. In a later chapter the practical application of the principles of management will be amplified.

For the purposes of explanation it is useful to divide the clinical picture into various aspects. In practical management the treatment of all aspects proceeds simultaneously. In this chapter the condition is considered under the following headings:

1. The spinal injury. The diagnosis and treatment of the damaged vertebral column and spinal cord it encloses. The assessment of the neurological damage.

2. The general condition. The management of the patient as a whole, the details of which are dictated by abnormal physiology consequent upon interruption of spinal cord function.

Again it must be reiterated that this division is artificial and that in practical management all aspects proceed together.

The aims of management of the spinal injury

1. To prevent further damage to the cord during first-aid measures, transport, diagnosis and subsequent nursing.
2. To aid healing of the damaged spine so that it can function effectively as a weight bearing organ whether the patient can stand or only sit and lie.
3. To relieve pressure on the cord.
4. To achieve healing of compound injuries after proper wound debridement and toilet.

The measures used to achieve these aims are similar to those in uncomplicated vertebral fractures but with certain exceptions, the most important of which is that plaster of Paris fixation in the form of jackets or beds is never used to support the spine below the site of the lesion where there is anaesthesia of the skin and deep tissues; sores would be inevitable, for the patient has no stimulus for complaint should the cast press unevenly over bony points where sensation is absent. Accordingly, unstable fractures must be protected from displacement by other means; skull traction is most useful in cervical cases; internal fixation with plates or wire is sometimes used at this and lower levels. Always the patient must be nursed in such a way that during all procedures the spine remains supported and its natural curves are preserved and the damaged parts are not allowed to displace. The demands of general management necessitate frequent shifting of the patient from one position to another; for this to be done safely, skill and experience are necessary. To achieve this, good techniques must be soundly learned and practised. Medical opinion still remains divided on many aspects of the management of cord injuries, and while controversial problems continue to be investigated, it is vital that whatever method is preferred by the medical team in charge, this should be pursued to the highest standard. Only by assiduous attention to detail in all respects can the merits of each method be assessed reliably.

Intelligent management of the general condition requires a knowledge of the abnormal physiology brought about by spinal cord injury. Most of what is to be explained refers to complete transections; occasional reference will be made, however, to differences when the lesion is incomplete.

The physiology of spinal cord injury

The results of complete transection of the spinal cord are:

1. Loss of voluntary movement below the level of the lesion. The

term *voluntary* must be included, for involuntary movement below the level of the spinal cord lesion is seen frequently. These movements can be stimulated by scratching or pinching the skin of the part, and they are outside the patient's control. Involuntary movement is occasionally responsible for a false sign of recovery, unless the observer is aware of the phenomenon. The loss may not be total in incomplete cord lesions.

2. Loss of sensation below the level of the lesion (often the patient believes he can feel the part, but this is completely subjective and he is oblivious of the examiner touching or pricking the skin). Similarly to movement, the loss of sensation may not be complete.
3. Loss of normal bladder control.
4. Loss of normal bowel control.
5. Loss of normal sexual function.
6. Loss of normal control of the sympathetic nervous system.

If the level of the lesion is below the first thoracic segment, the lower limbs and a variable amount of the trunk are affected and this is called *paraplegia.* When the level is higher and the upper limbs are involved, the condition is called *tetraplegia* (sometimes called quadriplegia). At one time, paraplegia was regarded as a difficult condition to treat; tetraplegia was hardly considered and it was thought better that such severely afflicted patients should die rather than pursue a fruitless and dismal life of chronic incapacity. Nowadays, tetraplegia has taken the place of paraplegia as being a difficult condition to treat; paraplegia is relatively simple and the great pioneers in this field have shown how happy and useful paraplegic patients can be made, provided all aspects of rehabilitation are good and vigorous. Tetraplegia likewise must no longer be regarded as 'a condition not to be treated.' Patients with even the highest lesions can be offered some sort of useful existence; never let it be said by a nurse that the patient would be better dead.

In addition to upper limb involvement, tetraplegia differs from paraplegia in another important respect: the sympathetic nervous system is paralysed in the former. It is largely through the sympathetic nerves that centres in the brain exercise control over the heart, blood pressure, temperature control and certain other important mechanisms. The sympathetic nerves travel with the segmental nerves of the thoracic region and it is evident that in lesions above the first thoracic segment, the entire sympathetic outflow will be deprived of its source of control in the brain.

Some results of this paralysis of sympathetic function which may seriously affect nursing are:

1. The blood pressure is labile. It may fall alarmingly if the patient is sat up too quickly and loss of consciousness can ensue. This is regained if he is laid flat.
2. The nasal passages become congested and mouth breathing,

with consequent drying of the pharyngeal and laryngeal mucosae, is common.

3. Low blood sugar, loss of appetite and liver failure can occur. Careful choice of diet may be necessary to persuade the patient to have an adequate intake.

4. Sometimes difficulty in swallowing and regurgitation are seen in the early stages.

5. In this country the patient's temperature in the early stages is usually low—indeed, a temperature of 37°C may represent a pyrexia in the tetraplegic patient. In warm climates, however, where the environmental temperature is above 37°C, hyperpyrexia can occur because sweating is deficient. These effects are due to loss of proper heat control so that the patient's temperature tends to follow that of the environment. Both hypopyrexia and hyperpyrexia can cause death. In hypopyrexia more heat is being lost from the body than is available within, because the heat-conserving mechanism has failed and there is no muscle contraction (normally manifest as shivering), one of the most potent forms of heat generation. Other sources of heat are from ingested food and metabolism, both of which may be deficient. In the tetraplegic patient, as the temperature falls, the chemical reactions of the body (metabolism) also slow down so that even less heat is produced and so fall of temperature is progressive until death occurs (this is precisely what occurs when a normal person is exposed to excessively low temperatures and dies from 'exposure'—he falls asleep). Thus it may be necessary to maintain the temperature artificially during the first days using a thermostatically controlled electric blanket—*never* hot water bottles. The rectal temperature must be charted at one-hourly intervals and maintained between 35° and 37°C (96° and 98·4°F).

As the level of the spinal lesion rises there comes a time when segments of origin of the phrenic nerve (cervical 3, 4 and 5) are involved and the diaphragm weakens. Assisted respiration may be essential. Many patients with such high injuries die from respiratory failure before reaching hospital. Abdominal distension in the early period is common and this impedes the action of the diaphragm even further by resisting its descent in inspiration.

Some of these features are illustrated diagrammatically in Figure 3.1.

The causes of death

Untreated or poorly treated cases of spinal cord injury always die from the effects of disordered physiology. *All complications of spinal cord injury can be responsible for the patient's death* and it is as well, therefore, to view each with appropriate seriousness. The complications tend to snowball and actually encourage each other. The nurse has a key part to play in their prevention, and the converse statement

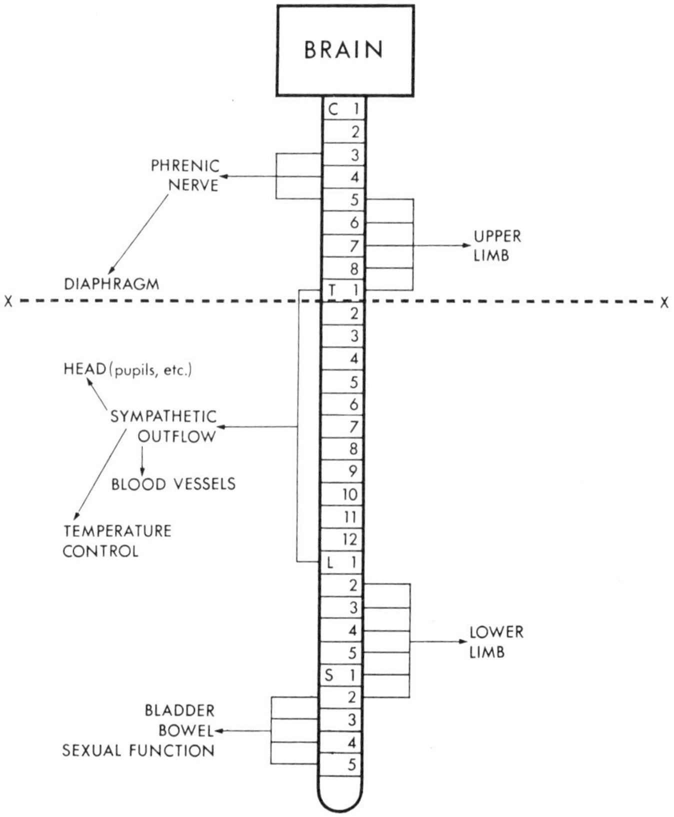

Fig. 3.1 The segments of origin of nerves supplying the limbs, diaphragm, bladder, bowel, sexual function and the sympathetic outflow. A lesion above the line X---X would cause tetraplegia; one below this level causes paraplegia.

is true—viz. poor nursing can precipitate complications, with frightening rapidity. The causes of death are summarised in Figure 3.2.

1. *Acute respiratory failure*

Acute respiratory failure may occur immediately, from paralysis of the diaphragm, or with dramatic suddenness during the first few days from exhaustion or increasing paralysis which can be due to upward extension of the swelling and bruising of the spinal cord. Again, should respiration be inadequate for one or another reason, carbon dioxide may be retained in the circulation and this may depress the controlling centres in the brain so that breathing becomes progressively more shallow.

Another cause of acute failure is regurgitation of stomach contents and their inhalation. This, coupled with the inability to cough effectively, results in the patient drowning. Coughing depends on forceful

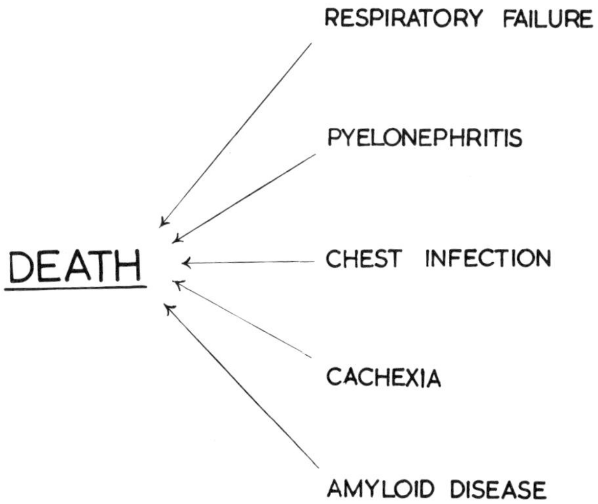

Fig. 3.2 The main causes of death consequent upon poorly treated spinal cord injuries.

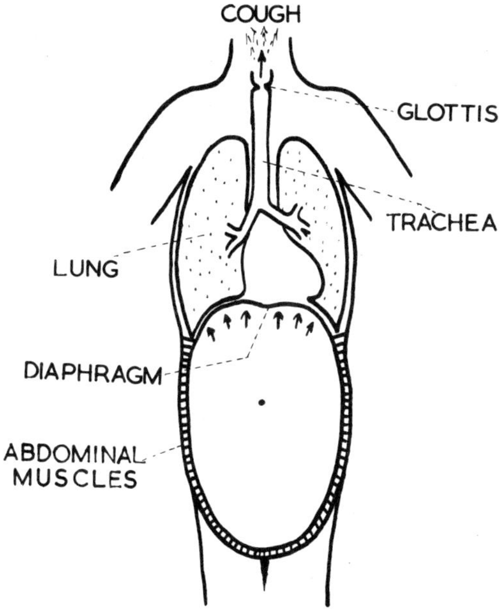

Fig. 3.3 Function of the abdominal muscles during coughing. Contraction of these drives the diaphragm upwards into the chest so that air is driven forcibly out of the lungs when the glottis opens.

expiration using the abdominal muscles to drive up the diaphragm, provided the diaphragm is contracting well so that satisfactory inspiration can occur; without the action of the abdominal muscles, coughing is weak. This weakness is marked in high paraplegia and tetraplegia (Fig. 3.3).

Principles of management. No patient with a high spinal lesion should be left alone during the acute period.

Facilities for suction, maintaining the airway, tracheostomy and access to medical assistance should be available all the time.

The nurse should be able to assist the patient in his coughing efforts by pressing on the upper abdomen firmly as he makes the attempt. This procedure is performed usually by the physiotherapist but she may not be readily available when the intelligent patient feels he wants to cough, and for this reason the nurse should be able to perform the simple manoeuvre shown in Figure 12.1

2. *Chronic respiratory failure*

Because of reduced ability to cough effectively, patients with tetraplegia and high paraplegia are prone to chest infection. The common cold can lead to very serious chest complications.

Principles of management. Assisted coughing, if prompt, may be the only therapy necessary. Thick sputum can be made manageable and more easily expectorated by inhalation of an aerosol, such as Alevaire. Antibiotics may be prescribed on medical advice, but are not without danger if prescribed indiscriminately in hospital.

Tracheostomy is occasionally necessary in the acute stages of high spinal cord injuries for the purposes of assisted respiration or aspiration of the bronchial tree by catheter suction. Patients with tracheostomy need to be nursed in the moistened air of a steam tent. A soft sterile catheter is used to suck out gently from the bronchial tree accumulating secretions. The tracheostomy tube and all accessible flanges should be cleaned carefully as necessary.

3. *Bladder dysfunction*

Immediately following injury to the spinal cord there is a period lasting from a few hours in partial lesions, to many weeks or even months in complete lesions, in which the segments of the cord below the injury are inactive. This is the period already referred to as the period of spinal shock. It is during this early period that the bladder losses all power to contract. The sphincters of the outlet remain tightly closed so that the bladder fills with urine and becomes very distended. Eventually, if unrelieved, the pressure of urine overcomes the resistance of the sphincter and urine overflows passively into the urethra while the bladder remains full and a reservoir of stagnant urine. This condition is sometimes referred to as retention with overflow and the stagnant urine easily becomes infected. Further, the raised pressure within the bladder can produce an obstruction to the flow of urine from the ureters and kidneys and they become progressively dilated (hydronephrosis). Again, if unrelieved, this condition leads to infection (pyelonephritis), as well as stone formation and destruction of kidney tissue. Whereas bladder dysfunction is the primary result of the paralysis it is the secondary effects which have serious and far reaching consequences for the patient. The secondary effects are common to both male and female patients alike but in the male the infections are more widespread because of the proximity and communication with the genital tract. Infection may spread to the prostate and seminal vesicles and to the epididymis and testis (epididymo-orchitis).

With the cessation of spinal shock a variety of modified types of bladder activity can become established. These depend not only on the particular type of cord and nerve injury but on the methods of treatment used to drain and train the bladder in the early stages. There is nearly always an imbalance between the power of bladder contraction and sphincter relaxation. This means that the bladder never empties and always contains some residual urine; this is a potential source of infection and stone formation.

Principles of management. (1) Preventing bladder distension and urine stagnation will reduce the risks of infection and preserve healthy kidney function. Catheterisation is performed according to some rigidly aseptic and atraumatic technique. The catheter may be left in the bladder (indwelling catheter) or it may be inserted and withdrawn after emptying the bladder at regular intervals throughout the day and night (intermittent catherisation). The choice of technique is a medical decision based on the clinical situation and the services available; (2) Preventing the urine from becoming over-concentrated is aided by a high fluid intake (3 l per 24 hours). Over-concentrated urine predisposes to the precipitation of solids and the formation of phosphatic debris and stones.

4. *Bowel dysfunction*

In the same way that the bladder becomes paralysed so do parts of the gastro-intestinal tract. In the initial period of spinal shock both the stomach and bowel can become grossly distended and inactive. This loss of activity is called paralytic ileus and it is a great source of danger to the patient. The stomach and intestine can become distended to the point of rupture and it is therefore absolutely imperative that the condition is recognised and treated as soon as possible. Diagnosis is a medical matter but the nurse can recognise the distended abdomen and the absence of bowel sounds.

Distension of the stomach and bowel can also embarrass the movement of the diaphragm and particularly in cases of cervical spinal cord injury. Poor inspiration leads to inefficient coughing and the bronchial tree cannot be cleared of its secretions.

The activity in the lower bowel and rectum returns to a greater or lesser extent after the cessation of the period of spinal shock. Nevertheless there is often a need to finger evacuate the rectal contents or to stimulate reflex action with the aid of rectal suppositories. Faecal mobility can be improved with the help of laxatives or aperients in appropriate doses.

Principles of management. Abdominal distension can be minimised by the passage of a flatus tube per rectum at regular intervals. Generalised paralytic ileus is relieved by the passage of a naso-oesophageal tube through which the stomach contents can be aspirated as required. If bowel sounds cannot be heard with a stethoscope it is often necessary to stop all fluids and solids by mouth and to administer fluids by intravenous infusions. Manual removal of accessible solid material becomes necessary when bowel motility returns and drives faeces into the lower rectum. Later, the rectum may empty in response to suppositories.

5. *Cachexia*

Cachexia is a syndrome of wasting of the tissues, general exhaustion and poor resistance to infection. It was seen regularly before the

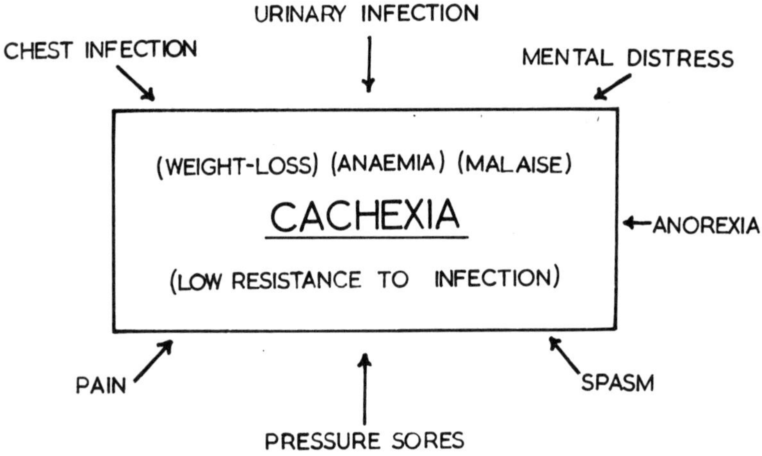

Fig. 3.4 The causes of cachexia consequent upon poorly treated spinal cord injuries.

modern treatment of spinal cord injuries was understood, and was due to recurrent urinary infection discussed above and the distressing triad of *pressure sores, spasm* and *pain* considered below. The causes of cachexia are depicted in Figure 3.4.

Pressure sores. Unlike paralysis from such a cause as poliomyelitis, patients with complete cord injuries lose all sensation below the level of the lesion and have no appreciation of the minor discomforts which make normal individuals change their position frequently, whether in bed, sitting, standing, or sleeping. Such discomforts occur when some part of the body has been subjected to pressure for more than an hour or two; the part is deprived of a satisfactory capillary blood supply and local nerves become irritable. If not relieved, the impaired blood supply results in cellular death, usually of the deeper tissues; the deep necrosis shows as an ominous dull red or purple flush and it is very fortunate if ulceration does not follow. (Pressure sores occur in the elderly, or in patients enfeebled from debilitative

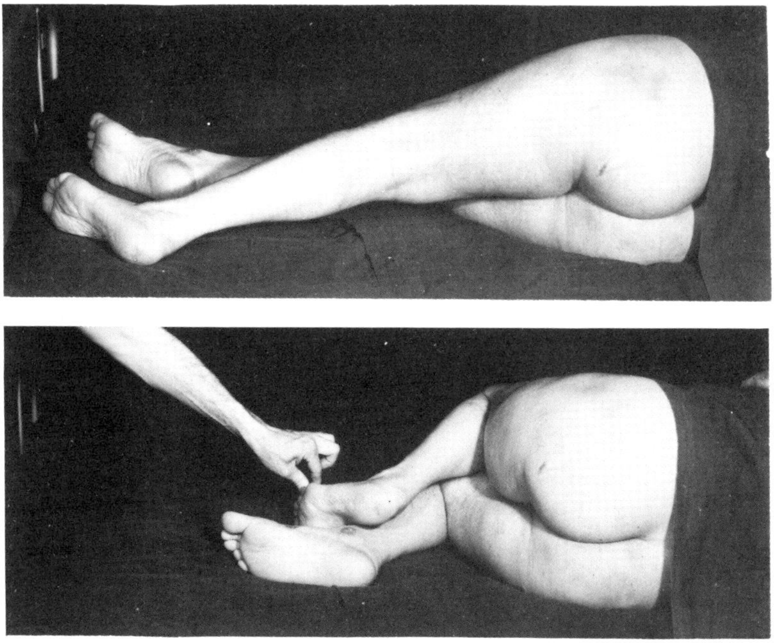

Fig. 3.5 The characteristic posture of flexion-adduction spasm affecting the lower limbs. The increased prominence of the sacrum, ischia, greater trochanters and knees is well seen. The knees are pressed together and nursing of the perineal area is difficult.

illness, partly because they are not sufficiently alert or strong to move themselves and partly because the general circulation is so poor.)

Inevitably, pressure sores become infected; they afford a constant drain of pus or exudate, fluids which are rich in protein. Protein is the raw material for cellular growth of all types including red blood cells, and for some of the defence mechanisms against infection; thus bed sores predispose to poor healing, anaemia, and secondary infection of the lungs and kidneys.

Spasm. Spasm is the name given to the involuntary sustained

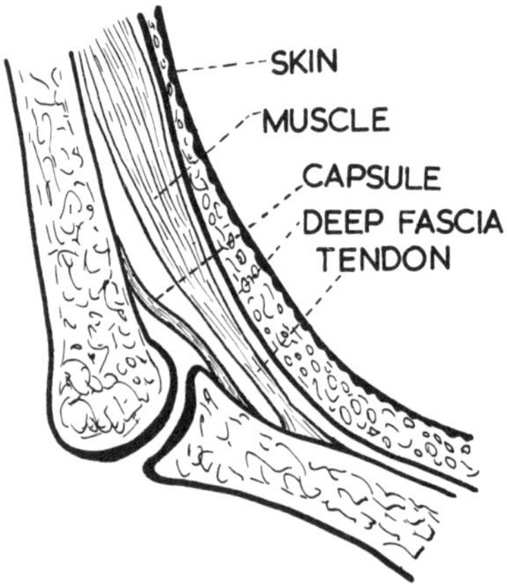

Fig. 3.6 The structures adjacent to a joint which if contracted would produce a contracture.

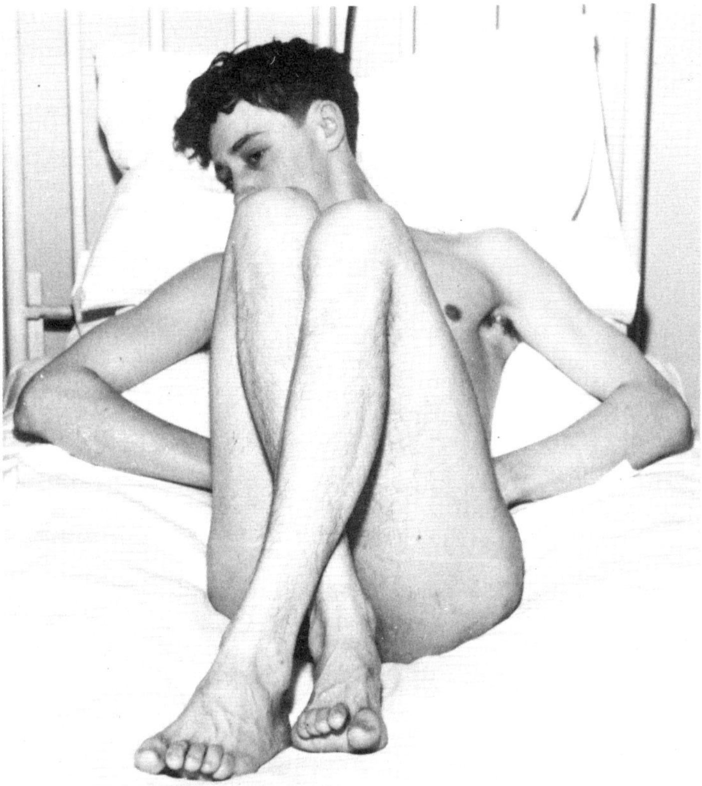

Fig. 3.7 Patient with severe flexion contractures at the hips and knees.

contraction of a muscle group. As a result, the joint or joints controlled by this muscle group are put into a position of deformity over which the patient has no control. Commonly, spasm affects several joints, and the limb may be held in characteristic positions. For example, in the lower limb, a common pattern is flexion and adduction of the hips, flexion of the knee and dorsiflexion of the foot (Fig. 3.5).

Spasm is a feature of the independent function of the lower isolated segment of the spinal cord below the level of the lesion. The general activity of this segment can be stimulated by almost any source of irritation in the lower part of the body. Such irritation is properly called afferent stimulation; a reflex arc is created and the spasm so caused constitutes its efferent component. The important examples of afferent stimuli are:

Sensory stimulation from a distended bladder
Sensory stimulation from a distended bowel
Sensory irritation from a pressure sore
Sensory irritation from contractures (see below)
Sensory irritation from bed clothes, wearing apparal or badly fitting appliances
Emotional upsets.

The return of reflex activity coincides with the cessation of spinal shock. It may take weeks or months for reflex activity to develop into the condition of spasm and much depends on the level and completeness of the spinal cord injury. Thus high lesions, as occur in injuries to the neck and upper dorsal spine, are particularly likely to develop reflex muscle spasms. Low lesions of ten remain relatively flaccid and less trouble to the patient. The intensity of spasm is very variable and great efforts must be made to minimise it. When spasm becomes dominant in one position it produces a shortening of muscles, joint capsules and ligaments. The passive range of movement of joint becomes limited and the condition is called a *contracture* (Fig. 3.6). When a contracture is stretched in an effort to regain the lost range of movement, the nerves in the shortened capsular ligaments and muscles are stimulated and further spasm is produced. Thus a contracture, once developed is likely to persist (Fig. 3.7). Contractures can become so severe that the affected joint may dislocate.

There are numerous patterns of spasms in spinal cord injuries. When the hips and knees are severely flexed the condition is sometimes referred to as 'paraplegia, in flexion'. When the hips and knees are extended and the feet plantar flexed the condition is called 'paraplegia in extension'.

Paraplegia in extension is more commonly seen in incomplete spinal cord lesions. Very occasionally there is flexion in one limb and extension in another.

Spasm and voluntary movement exist together in some incomplete lesions. When this occurs voluntary movements appear laboured and stiff; they are said to be spastic.

Spasm can occur in many neurological diseases but it is especially serious in paraplegia or tetraplegia because of the danger of pressure sore formation. As has been stated, pressure sores occur over bony points, and in the common flexor pattern of spasm these areas are thrown into even greater prominence, viz. the sacrum, ischia, trochanters, knees and heels.

Sometimes spasm is painful, the patient suffering severe cramp-like sensations; again, but not always, this state of affairs occurs in incomplete cord lesions. Because of pain and the associated involuntary movements, the patient may be unable to rest and quickly becomes exhausted.

Briefly, it may be stated that spasm is not a direct cause of death but affords a potent aggravation of all other complications. Further, it is stimulated by any irritation, e.g. sores, bladder infection and contractures. Prevention lies in avoidance of these afferent sources (Fig. 3.8).

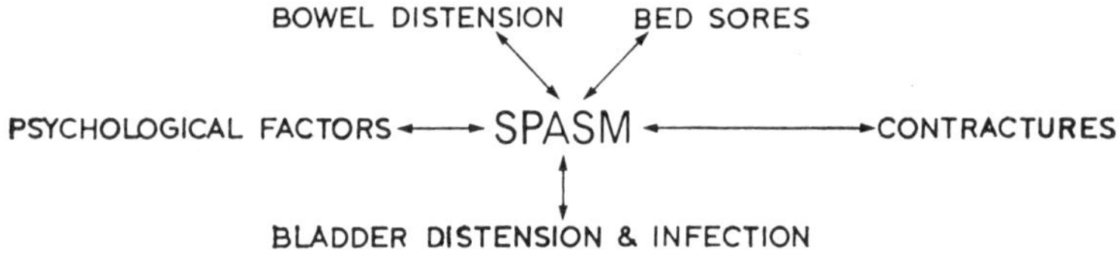

Fig. 3.8 The causes of spasm.

Pain. Several types of pain occur in spinal cord injuries:

a. *Painful spasm*—which has been described above.

b. *Root pain*, due to irritation of nerves at the site of injury. This is often felt as a band round the body and may be aggravated by movement.

c. *Diffuse, ill-defined pain.* Once established, this is a very difficult type of pain to treat. It is thought to arise partly in the proximal stump of the cord at the site of injury, and may take on any modality, such as a diffuse ache, tingling, burning, etc. Phantom phenomena are often mixed with the pain; for example, the patient thinks he can feel his lower limbs and sometimes believes he is actually moving them, or worse, they are moving themselves. Sometimes the limbs feel abnormal in shape and length and patients become very distressed. Curiously, this particular type of pain and sensation are, in part, under psychological control, and if the patient's attention can be diverted from them by interesting activities, the phenomena may disappear. Nevertheless, patients must never be told they are imagining their discomforts; there is nothing more demoralising than to be told this. Their pain is very real to them. If the pain is treated by giving strong analgesics (only drugs producing mental relaxation such as morphine increasingly high dosage. Drug addiction used to be common.

Figure 3.9 shows the inter-relating factors which contribute to the decline of the paraplegic or tetraplegic patient and it becomes plain that there exists a series of inter-relating vicious circles. Unless all of these are prevented, rehabilitation will be impossible. Further, it should be most evident that *prevention is better than cure,* and it must

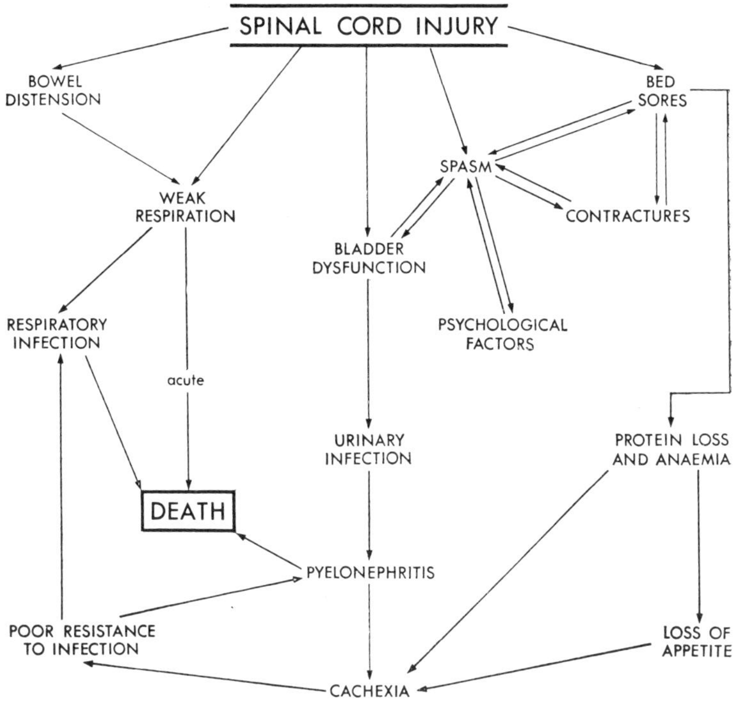

Fig. 3.9 The 'vicious circles' consequent upon spinal cord injury.

be reiterated that in no field does the nurse exercise so much control over the patient's future. Mistakes made in the early days are frequently irrevocable.

Psychological aspects

Immediately after spinal cord injury, it is usual for the uninformed patient to be completely unaware of the seriousness of his plight. Although he cannot move the limbs below the level of the cord lesion, he believes that they move and that he can feel them albeit imperfectly: the parts seem somehow unreal. The possibilities of permanent paralysis and loss of sensation, let alone the significance of bowel and bladder dysfunction, are not appreciated; commonly, completely tetraplegic patients are unable to believe that senseless hands are their own until they trace visually their forearms and arms to the shoulders which they are able to feel. This event, or some comparable revelation, comes as a catastrophic shock. Other features of the condition have to be assimilated successively and this process culminates in a suspicion or some knowledge of the possible or probable permanency of the interruption of cord function. The rate at which this information is fed verbally to the patient must be controlled by the doctor in charge of the case and no other person; the doctor uses his discretion and experience in judging each individual capacity. He may conclude that a particular patient can never be told his true prognosis while another person must be given a definite answer to the question: 'Will I get better?' Not all lesions are permanent and many improve or recover; much experience is necessary before a prognosis of value can be advised. In the case of a permanent deficit, it is usual for the door to hope to be allowed to close very slowly in order that the patient may have time to adjust mentally. Despite this lingering possibility of hope, the average patient is despondent and needs reassurance from all who come into contact with him, especially nurses, his constant companions during the early period. The aim is to let him know that, despite the gravity of the situation, he is still of value to the community and his family. This aim is achieved by example, demeanour and interest on the part of all concerned. Words of pity and sorrow have no place; it must be made clear that the patient himself has something to give and a duty to make the most of what nervous function remains. Usually, it is of value to point out that things could have been worse, e.g. the paraplegic patient could have been rendered tetraplegic, and the level in a tetraplegic patient could have been higher so that 'that vital function of the biceps would have been lost.' Statements to the effect that the patient might have been killed must be avoided, however, because in the early stages patients sometimes agree that this would have been better and a verbal battle for hope is lost. Without satisfactory mental adjustment, all other efforts to treat the physical aspects of the condition are wasted. This unhappy state can occur so easily.

To illustrate this statement, consider the plight of the young man reduced by injury from being the breadwinner and head of his family to being its most dependent member. Usually, he can no longer perform his original work; his earning power fails, he has to tolerate the embarrassment of bladder and bowel management and he can no longer reproduce; neither can be play actively with children he may already possess, nor indulge in the vast number of common activities which we take for granted. It is easy for him to feel utterly despondent, unwanted, and no use to anyone.

In high tetraplegia, this plight reaches its zenith, for the patient may be reduced to what is virtually a living head. And yet, this head contains a marvellous brain with facilities for thinking, seeing, hearing, smelling and talking. Further, the mind has memories, mental skills and, above all, feelings and emotions. Provided there is some channel for voluntary movement, although this may be from only the mouth, modern medico-mechanical devices can alleviate to a variable degree the state of dependence, even in the most grossly disabled case.

The nurse has great responsibilities in this field for, during day-to-day contact with the patient, her attitude may decide whether or not he can find any degree of happiness again; impatience, disgust or lack of interest can easily filter through to the sensitive invalid and these must be guarded against. The nurse always appears *interested*; this may require enormous effort. Any person unable to act in this way should keep away from severely handicapped people. Of course, it is not only the nurses who are important in these respects; all personnel, orderlies, physiotherapists, maids, occupational therapists, doctors and, very important, relatives, exercise effect over the patient's morale.

So frequently, it is the small things which require vigilance. For example, it is degrading to be referred to as a 'para' or a 'tetra,' or a 'T.9 lesion'; 'The patient is Mr Jones, who sustained a fracture of the ninth thoracic vertebra last Tuesday,' takes longer to say, but gives back some identity and status which Mr Jones stands in danger of losing.

Non-traumatic lesions of the spinal cord

Because spinal cord dysfunction has such widespread skeletal and visceral effects, patients with disease of the cord other than trauma are frequently looked after in spinal injury centres. The nurse is required to care for all aspects of the case.

As has been explained, many systems of the body are affected secondarily by spinal cord disease and it is for this reason that these conditions are different from, for example, the relatively simple paralysis of poliomyelitis. In both traumatic and non-traumatic lesions, the interruption of cord function may be *complete* or *incomplete*. In incomplete lesions there is some sparing of cord function; for example, sensation may be preserved but there is no voluntary movement below the level of the damage; or motor function may be severely impaired in the upper limbs but relatively good in the lower limbs. In complete lesions there is no sparing of motor or sensory function.

Common types of spinal cord lesions may be classified as follows:

Congenital

Spina bifida. The baby is born with incomplete closure of the spinal canal. Apart from the neurological deficit, there may be a tuft of hair at the site or, in severe cases, a leakage of cerebro-spinal fluid; it can occur at any level but is usually lumbar or sacral. In minor cases, symptoms may not appear until late childhood.

Deformities

Scoliosis. Progressive scoliosis can sometimes cause paraplegia. The cause of the scoliosis may be congenital or acquired (e.g. poliomyelitis) or idiopathic (i.e. cause unknown).

Kyphosis. This may be congenital (e.g. hemivertebra) or acquired (e.g. tuberculosis of a vertebral body with collapse).

Degenerations

Multiple sclerosis. Scattered destruction and scarring of areas of the cord and brain. The cause is unknown.

Transverse myelitis. A segment of cord is destroyed and replaced by a scar. The cause may be a virus infection.

Cervical spondylosis. Degenerative bony changes in the cervical spine cause pressure on the cord.

Vascular

Arteriosclerotic myelopathy. Usually affects the cervical cord; blood supply is progressively impaired and a segment of cord dies.

Haematomyelia. Bleeding within the substance of the cord; this is sometimes spontaneous but may be due to trauma.

Infective

Tuberculous meningitis. May affect the membranes covering both brain and spinal cord.

Pott's parapelgia. As mentioned above, tuberculosis may affect the vertebral bodies causing collapse and a kyphos.

Tumours

Primary. Tumours may develop in the cord, from the meninges or from the bone of the vertebral column.

Secondary carcinoma. More common than primary tumours; usually arises in a vertebra; common primary sources are breast, lung, prostate, kidney and thyroid.

None of these causes of non-traumatic spinal cord disease is very common.

It should be noted that in any condition where there is loss of cutaneous or deep sensation, special nursing cares of the types to be described may be necessary. Examples other than spinal cord disease are: polyneuritis, in which there is loss of function in peripheral nerves, and traumatic division of large peripheral nerves. Again, in cases of severe muscular weakness (e.g. muscular dystrophy, in which the muscles lose all power to contract) and in elderly, feeble patients, the same special nursing care is required.

4. The Nursing Management of the Whole Patient

Success lies in the *prevention* of complications, and in this concept the one chance of really successful management. This is because, once allowed to develop, all the great complications tend to perpetuate themselves. For example:

1. *Pressure sores* can, it is true, be persuaded to heal, but the skin cover so obtained is unstable and scarred; this predisposes to further ulceration from relatively minor trauma (Fig. 4.1).
2. *Spasm,* if allowed to continue, will lead to formation of joint contractures which themselves stimulate more spasm.
3. *Urinary infection* damages the bladder lining and long standing and recurrent infections lead to scarring.

Scarring occurs at the bladder outlet and in the bladder wall both of which become markedly thickened. This makes reflex and straining micturition more inefficient; there may be a return to the state of retention with overflow which may produce back pressure on the kidneys and, even more serious, infection in the kidney tissues.

Chronic infections also predispose to stone formation and complications in the male genitalia.

4. *Malnutrition and anaemia,* once established, are often responsible for anorexia (poor appetite). The reduced resistance to infection potentiates disease of the urinary tract and chest, sores are more likely and all of these make the patient feel ill and even less willing to take nourishment.
5. *Despondency,* due to poor psychological management, is a potent inhibitor of the will to fight the new difficulties of life; less and less interest is taken in survival.

The reader's attention is directed again to the scheme outlined in Figure 3.9 which demonstrates how the complications are interrelated, sometimes provoking each other and forming a series of vicious circles.

The main aim of good nursing is, therefore, the prevention of the complications. It should be frankly recognised that should complications occur, it is due usually to some breach in technique, and even more strenuous efforts will be required if the inherent vicious circles are to be broken.

The theory of the specialised nursing is easily understood but the practice is often difficult. One reason for this difficulty is that the demands on nursing man-power, even for one patient with a spinal cord injury, are so lavish. Many hospitals just do not have the staff available; it need be no reflection on their goodwill and nursing capability that attempts to look after the occasional patient fail. In a spinal injuries centre the routine procedures are already established and the inevitable problems of management can be overcome from previous experiences. *Whenever possible, patients with spinal cord injuries should be transferred to special units at once.* The work of such units is made manifestly more difficult if complications have been allowed to ensue. In Great Britain, difficulty in transfer to specialised units rarely presents, unless there are other complicating injuries precluding transport, but in some countries immediate transfer may be impossible, and the patient must be cared for, if only temporarily, in the general hospital.

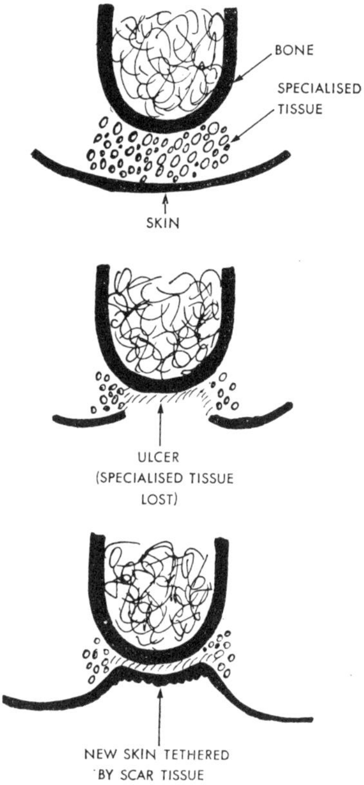

Fig. 4.1 The formation and healing of a pressure sore over a bony prominence (e.g. ischial tuberosity). The thin resultant scar is prone to further ulceration due to loss of specialised weight-bearing tissues.

In the next chapters, various aspects of management are considered

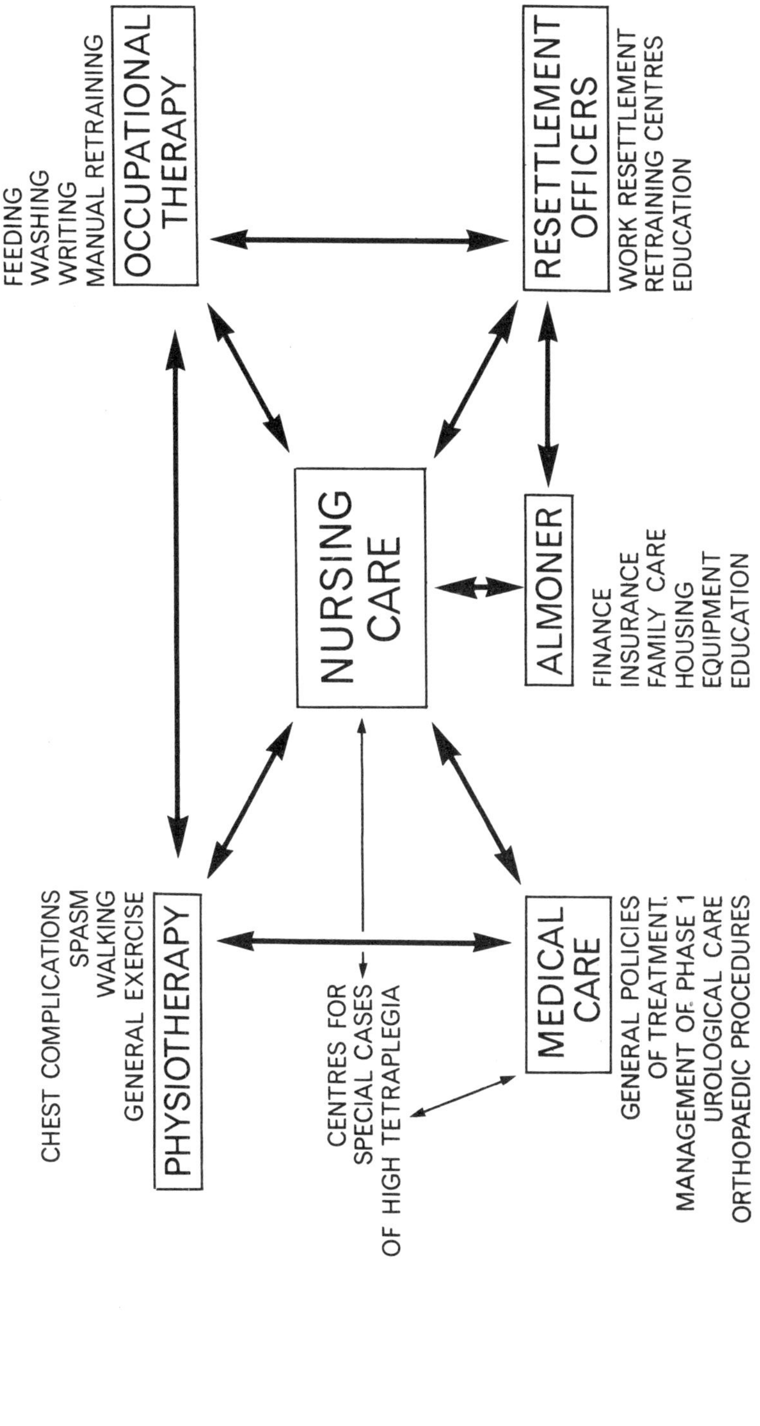

Fig. 4.2 The nurses' central position in the organised management of spinal cord injuries.

and actual techniques described. The details do not purport to be the only methods for successful management, but the underlying principles are accepted generally.

Each section is concerned with the *prevention* of complications and is entitled with this in mind.

It is stressed for the last time that the nursing management is the hub on which depend all other aspects of treatment; on the other hand, the nurse's efforts will be worth while only if she understands the outline of aims and methods employed by other departments and co-operates with them (Fig. 4.2).

5. The Prevention and Treatment of Pressure Sores

The skin and subcutaneous tissues in the anaesthetic and paralysed areas are liable to breakdown at any time but never more so than in the first hours and days after spinal cord injury. All areas must be protected from abrasions and prolonged pressure and this can only be achieved by regular changes of position. It is also during the same time that the injured spine requires its most careful handling and accordingly a reliable turning routine is absolutely vital. There must be an adequate number of trained staff available to lift and turn a patient with a well rehearsed and gentle routine at *two hourly intervals* throughout *the day and night*. If this is not done the nursing management will fail. The intervals may be lengthened only when the skin circulation improves and the tolerance to pressure increases. Each time a patient is turned the skin of the areas on which he last lay is examined in a good light for evidence of excessive *redness, discoloration* or *induration* which are the warning signs of impending pressure necrosis.

The turning routines may vary but the principles remain the same irrespective of any special apparatus that may be used in conjunction with them. Patients should be lifted, not dragged, and great care taken to support and position the paralysed limbs in their natural anatomical alignments.

Patients with spinal cord injuries should be transferred as soon as possible to special units where they can benefit from the collective expertise of the staff and facilities so essential for their comprehensive care. An example of a sacral sore is shown in Figure 5.1; the nurses attempting to look after this patient, who was very ill after his injury, did their best but were too few in number.

There will be occasions, however, when for some reason a patient cannot be transferred to a spinal injuries unit and, at the same time, the large number of staff required for manual turning is not available. It is in these circumstances that the Stryker frame is of value; with the aid of this device, patients can be turned from the supine position to the prone position by one person. Frequently, the fully prone position is not tolerated easily, especially in the presence of respiratory difficulties, but with care and encouragement adaptation does occur. It is of most use in cervical injuries and is easily combined with skull traction. The Stryker frame does not replace nursing care; it makes it easier but should be regarded as a second-best method of treatment.

Other types of beds are available for use in routine or complicated situations: The Stoke Mandeville Egerton bed is used routinely at Stoke Mandeville Hospital (Fig. 5.2); the electrically operated Keane Roto Rest bed (Fig. 5.3) is of value for heavy patients or in those

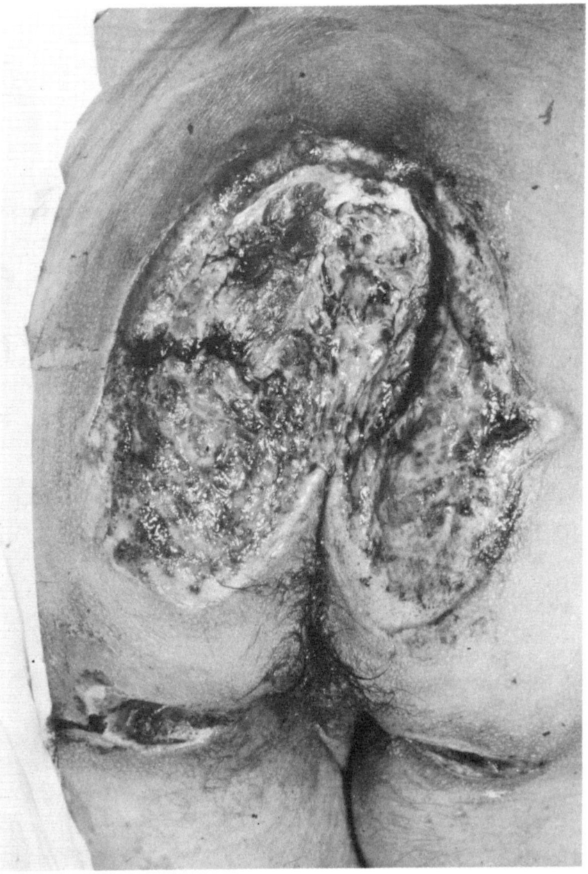

Fig. 5.1 A large sacral pressure sore.

with multiple injuries; other situations can be managed satisfactorily with pillow packs (Fig. 5.4) or on special frames (Fig. 5.5).

Ripple beds are common adjuncts to good nursing (Fig. 5.6); never allow this device to lull the nurse into a false sense of security. Only the assiduous turning care and meticulous inspection will prevent pressure sores in these patients.

The details of these nursing techniques are shown pictorially in Figures 5.7 and 5.8. Modifications vary from hospital to hospital, but the principles remain unchanged.

As healing of the vertebral fracture progresses, the time will arrive

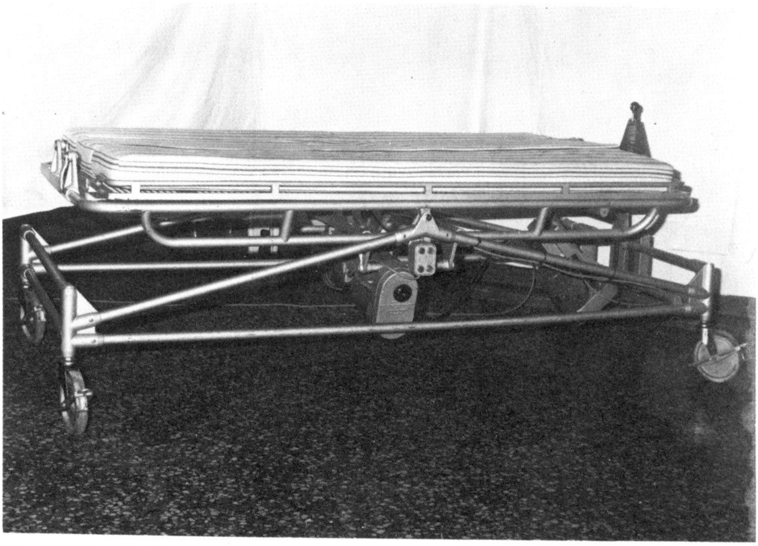

Fig. 5.2 Electrically operated Stoke Mandeville Egerton bed.

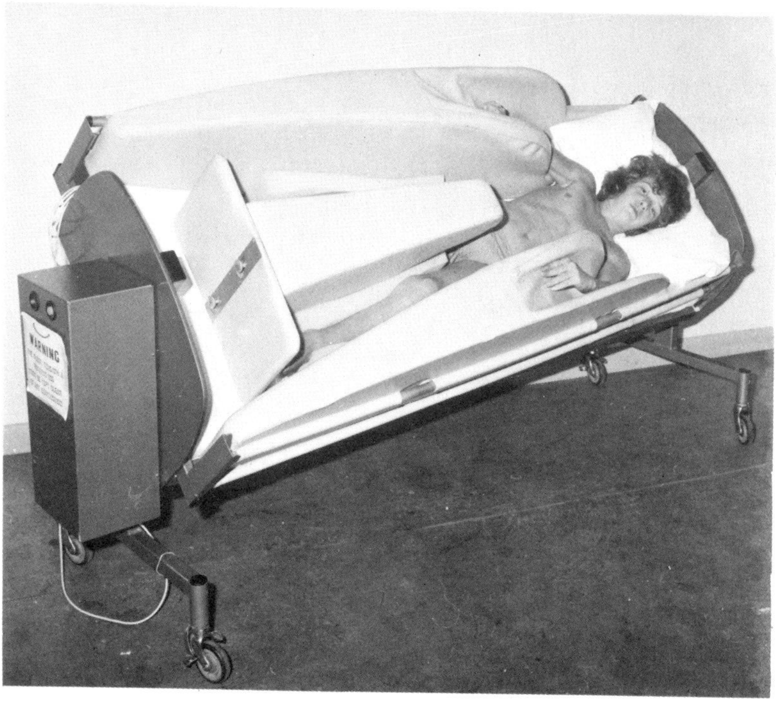

Fig. 5.3 Electrically operated Keane Roto Rest bed. This rotates from side to side automatically every fifteen minutes.

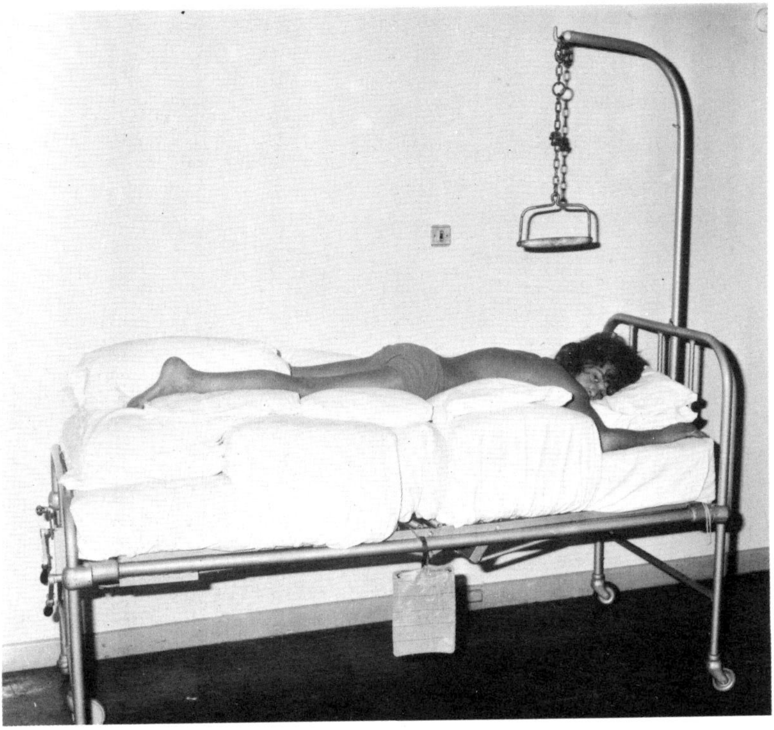

Fig. 5.4 Patient lying prone on pillow packs.

when the patient can help his nurses in turning routines (Fig. 5.9). The amount of effort safe for him to make will be judged on medical grounds; even patients with tetraplegia can assist to advantage (Fig. 5.10). Paraplegic patients otherwise fit will be taught by the nurses and physiotherapists to get out of bed unaided (Fig. 5.11).

Pressure sores occur not only in bed but in other circumstances; for example, pressure sores of the ischial tuberosities from prolonged sitting in one position. These are avoided as described in Chapter 12 by regularly relieving pressure on these areas. Similarly, sharp or angular articles in trouser pockets, projections in chairs and crumbs or other objects in the bed may cause damage to the anaesthetic skin surfaces. Other types of trauma are burns from cigarettes held in anaesthetic hands, scalds from hot bath water and the unwise use of hot water bottles.

A summary of the causes of pressure sores is given in Figure 5.12.

The treatment of pressure sores

The onset of a sore is heralded by a dark flush in the affected area; this is a sterile inflammation due to irritation from underlying tissues

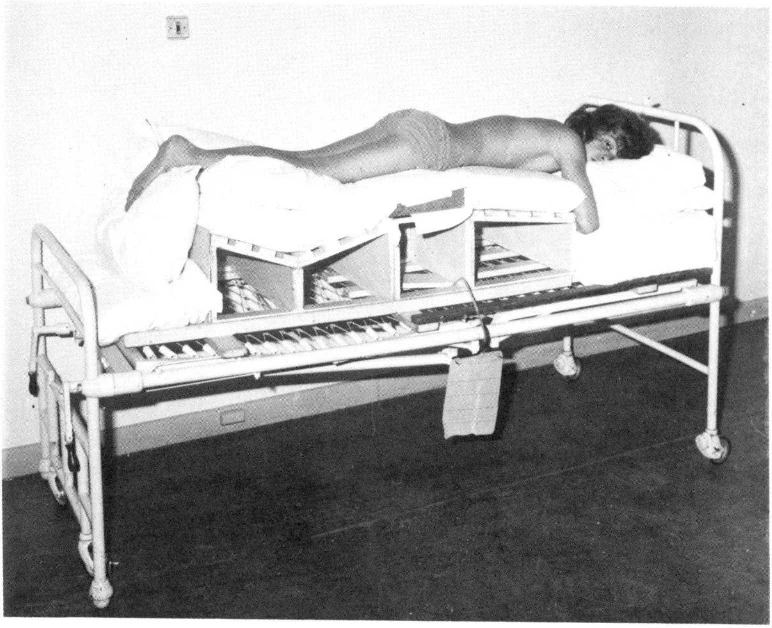

Fig. 5.5 Patient lying prone on Lodge Moor frame.

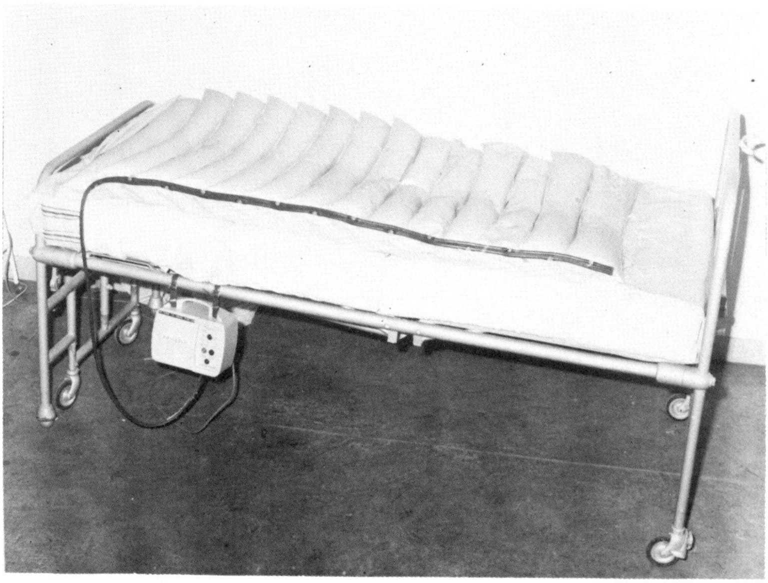

Fig. 5.6 A large celled matress with control unit.

Figure 5.7

Method for turning the paraplegic and tetraplegic patient. The photographs A to H demonstrate turning from the supine to the left lateral position; the procedures in turning from left lateral to right lateral, and right lateral back to the supine position, are simply extensions of the technique to be described. Figs. I and J show some modifications necessary in tetraplegia. During the first few weeks, turning must be performed with meticulous care. Later, as healing of the vertebral injury progresses, the patient is able to assist the nurses, subject to the extent of his paralysis. Paraplegic patients can eventually turn themselves, using a monkey chain.

The regime of turning is rigid and takes priority to most other ward duties. On each occasion, the patient is inspected for signs of pressure, and the bed for crumbs and other solid objects, which would prove injurious, should they lie under or even against him. Bed linen is of best quality and is renewed as necessary.

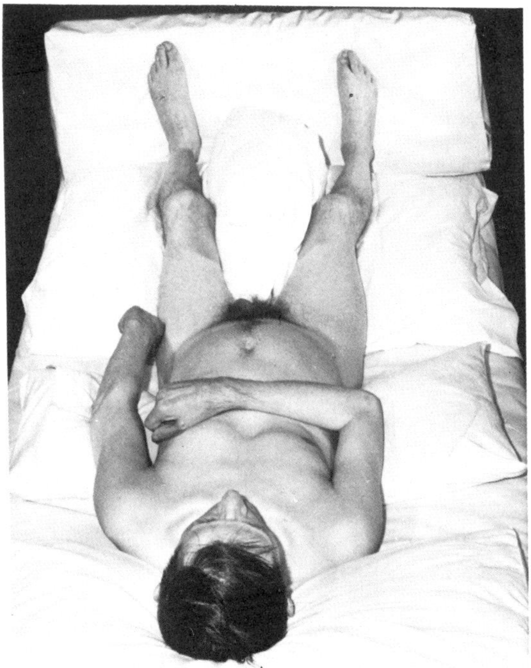

A

Fig. 5.7A and Fig. 5.7B, The patient lying supine. The lumbar curve is maintained by a flat pillow; this pillow is used as a support in subsequent alterations of the patient's position. In paraplegia there is no need for special positioning of the arms which are not paralysed nor anaesthetic. The lower limbs are supported in full, but relaxed extension, by more pillows. The hips are slightly abducted.

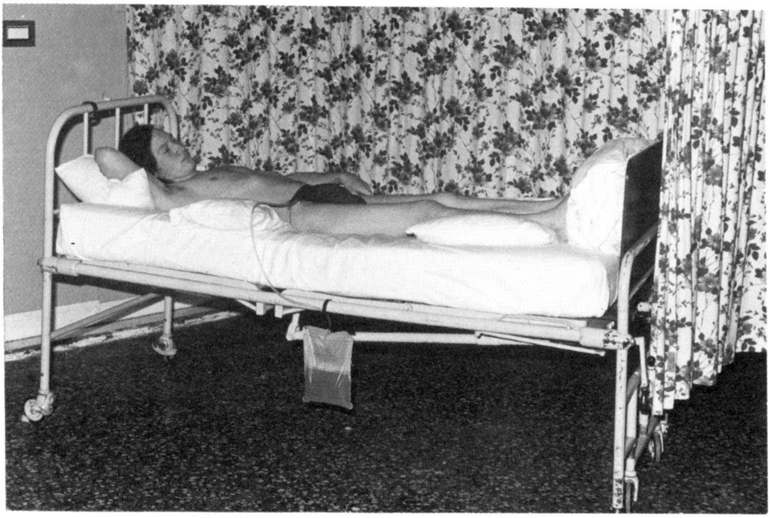

B

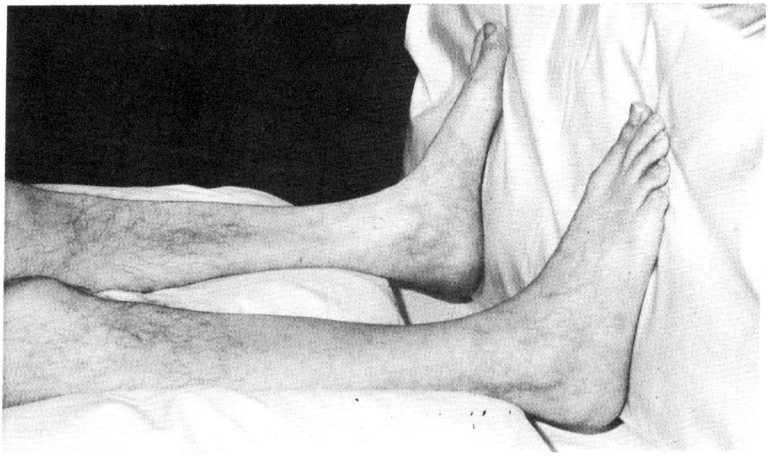

Fig. 5.7C, In the supine position the backs of the heels are spared all pressure, and the feet are supported in the neutral position by firm blocks of sorbo rubber, or biscuits of suitable size.

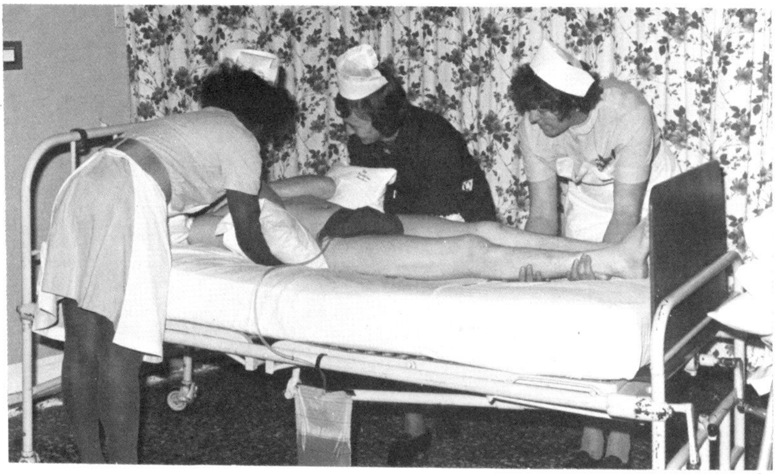

Fig. 5.7D, Nursing routine. First movement: lift to side of bed. In preparation for turning the patient from the supine to the left lateral position, all except the lumbar and head pillows are removed.

Using the lumbar pillow to advantage, two nurses, one on each side, slide their hands and forearms under the patient's trunk so as to provide evenly distributed support. A third nurse supports the lower limbs. If the patient has an indwelling catheter, particular care is taken to ensure that the drainage tube and connections are not pulled or dragged during the positioning of the patient.

At a given signal, the patient is lifted and moved smoothly to the side of the bed together with the lumbar pillow.

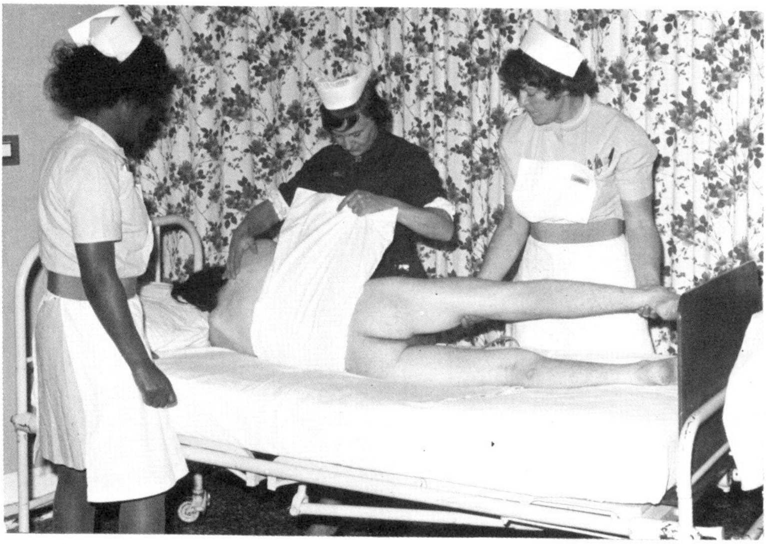

Fig. 5.7E, Nursing routine. Second movement: roll into the lateral position. The patient is rolled on to his side using the lumbar pillow while the upper leg is supported by another nurse.

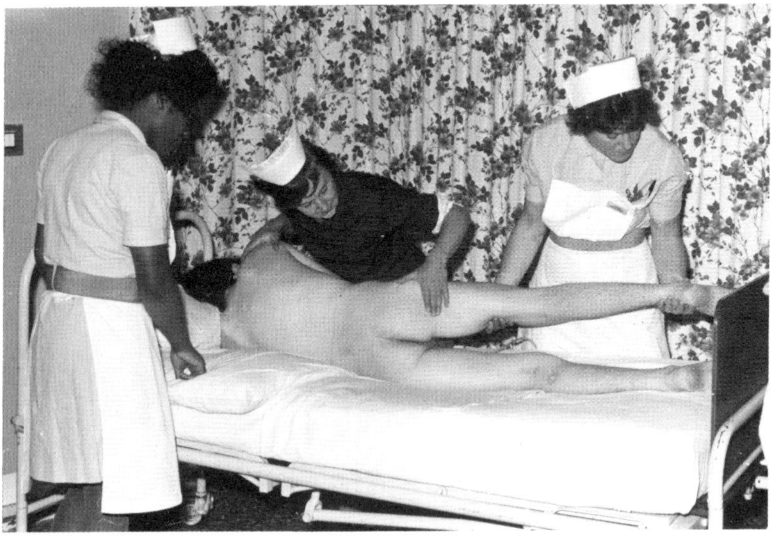

Fig. 5.7F, Nursing routine. Third movement: skin inspection. The lumbar pillow is laid flat on the bed so that the skin of the back, the buttocks, the upper hip, the heels and the ankles can be meticulously inspected by the nurses from their various positions. The pelvis and shoulders are supported throughout as shown.

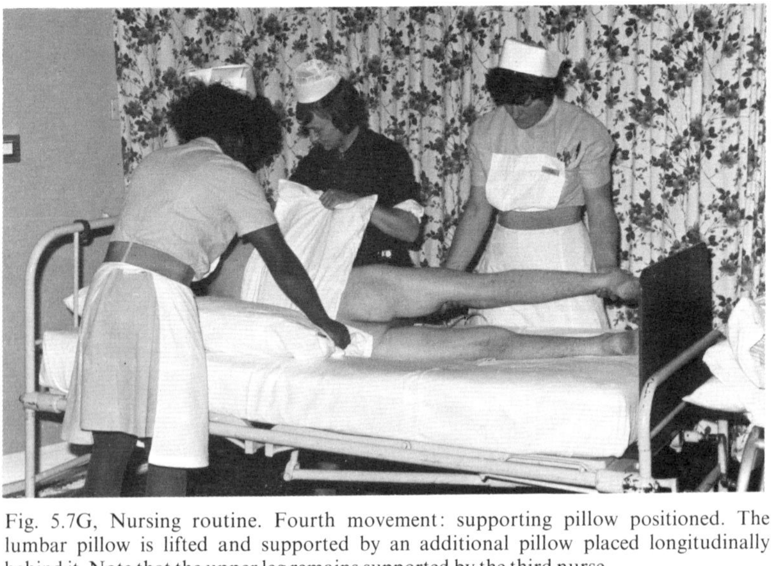

Fig. 5.7G, Nursing routine. Fourth movement: supporting pillow positioned. The lumbar pillow is lifted and supported by an additional pillow placed longitudinally behind it. Note that the upper leg remains supported by the third nurse.

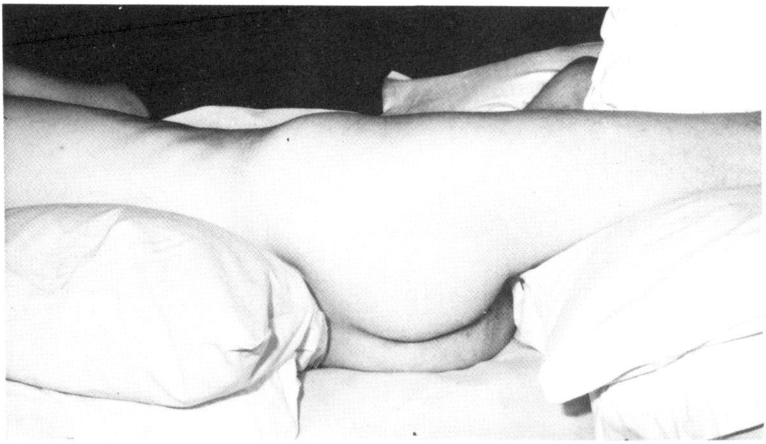

H

Fig. 5.7H and Fig. 5.7I, A close up view of the final position showing the back supported and the right buttock now clear of the bed; the upper leg is supported on additional pillows.

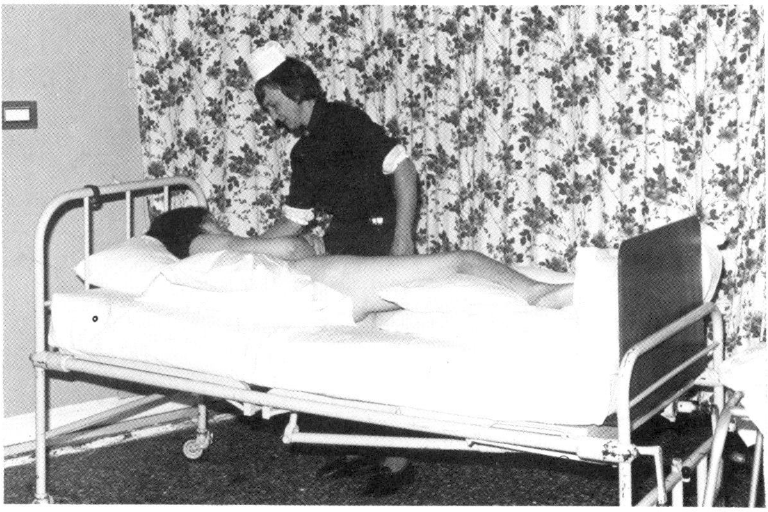

I

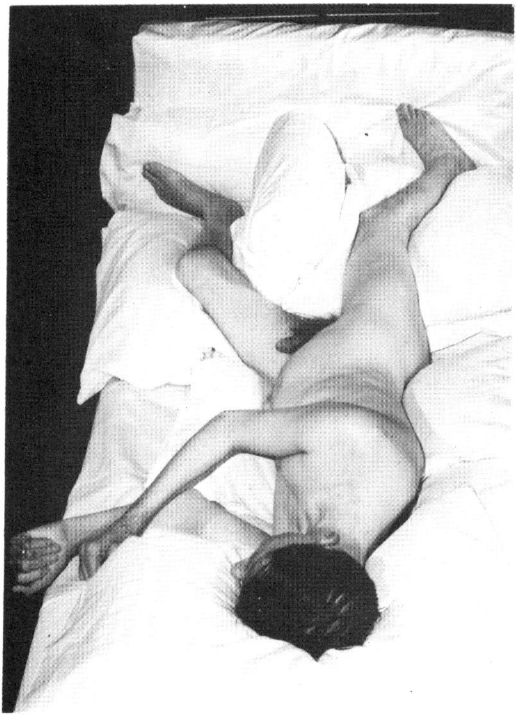

Fig. 5.7J, The completed left lateral position. The curves of the spine are preserved in normal alignment; the right lower limb is almost fully extended at the knee and the left one is flexed. In the paraplegic patient no special positioning of the upper limbs is required.

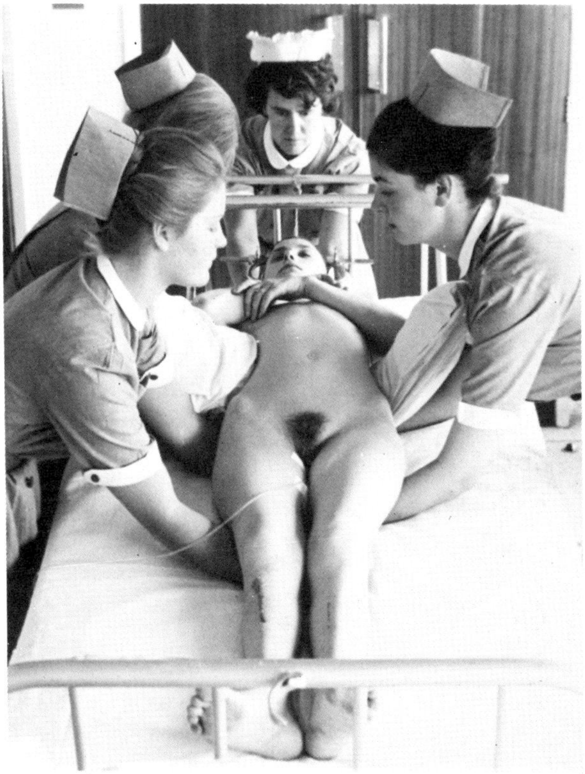

Fig. 5.7K, When turning a tetraplegic patient, a fourth nurse is required, the senior member of the team, who controls the patient's head and neck. She ensures that during all manoeuvres the head maintains its normal alignment with the shoulders. Before any change of position, she takes care that the traction system is not likely to be fouled by the bed head, and it is she who gives the command to perform the actual movement of the patient.

In the presence of severe upper limb paralysis, the arms must be controlled by tucking them in the lumbar pillow alongside the patient's body; this lumbar pillow is used in the tetraplegic case as a means of controlling the paralysed trunk. Reference to shows how the patient's head may be supported on a rolled towel; alternatively, an excavated sorbo rubber block may be used for this purpose. Further comparison with Fig. 2.27 shows the advantage of using a special traction unit which allows ease of access to the patient's head and neck during the turning procedure.

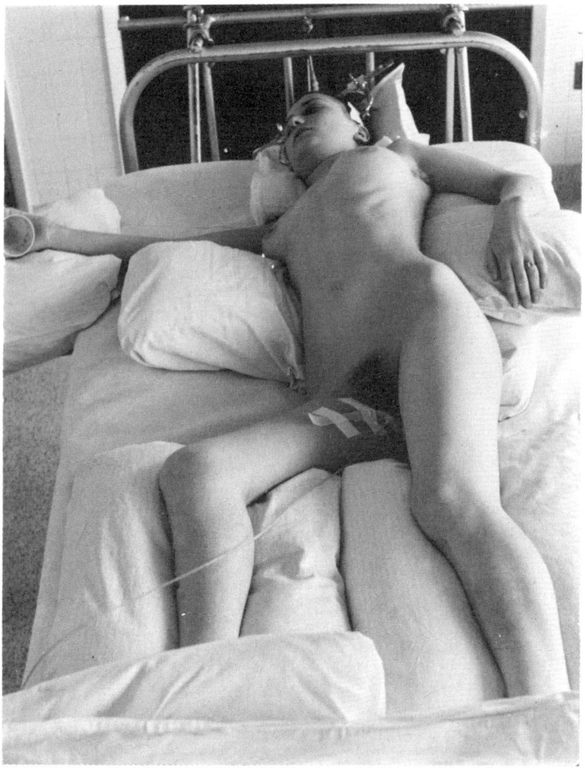

Fig. 5.7L, In addition to the lower limbs, the upper limbs of tetraplegic patients require careful positioning. The lower shoulder should be protected from bearing too much weight when in the lateral position, by placing the lumbar pillow fairly high. The lower elbow should lie comfortably extended and the fingers allowed to curl loosely round some sizeable object, so that they do not remain passively flexed for long periods. The upper arm may be positioned in the manner shown, or may lie across the body on another pillow; it should not rest directly on the chest. Bedclothes should be light and not impede respiration.

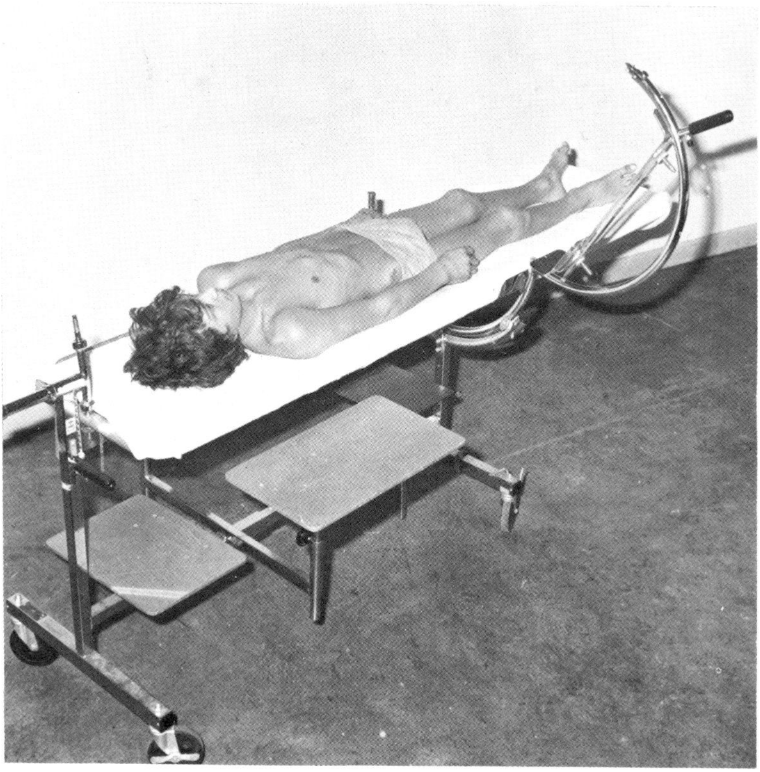

Fig. 5.8A, Patient lying supine on a Stryker Frame. This provides a means of turning a patient from the supine to the prone position when few nurses are available. During the change of position the patient lies sandwiched between two stretchers, the upper one of which is removed after turning; the stretchers rotate between a pivot at the head end and a circular clamp at the other. The apparatus is freely mobile on wheels.

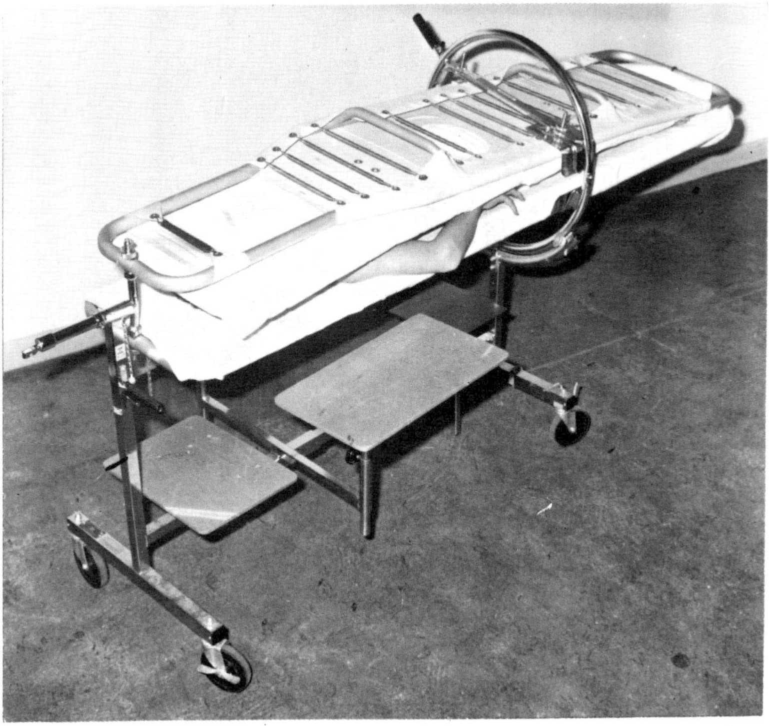

Fig. 5.8B, The upper stretcher has been applied preparatory to turning the patient from the supine to the prone position. Note the clamp which replaces straps used in earlier models of the Stryker frame.

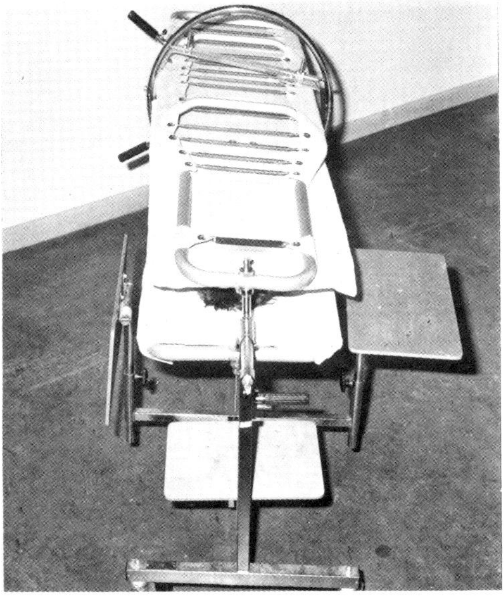

Fig. 5.8C, The clamp is closed securely.

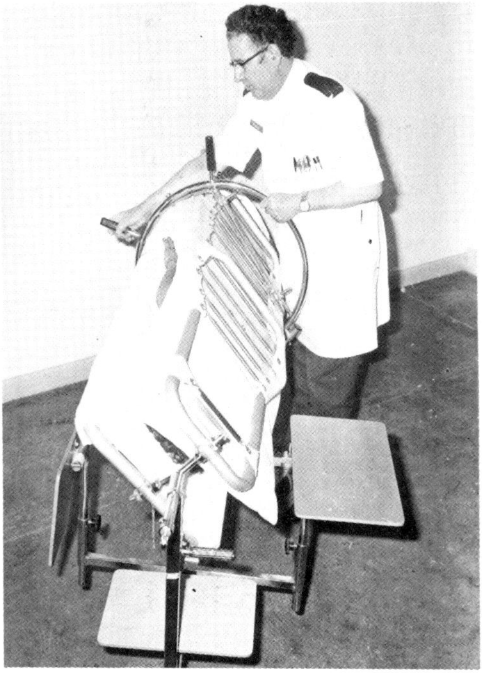

Fig. 5.8D, The closed clamp is used as the turning mechanism. It can be operated easily by one nurse.

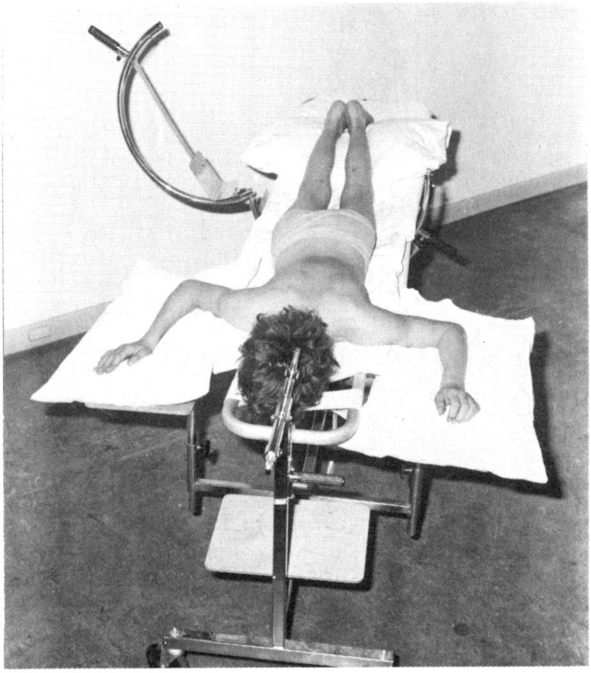

Fig. 5.8E, The turn completed, the upper stretcher is removed after unlocking the clamp.

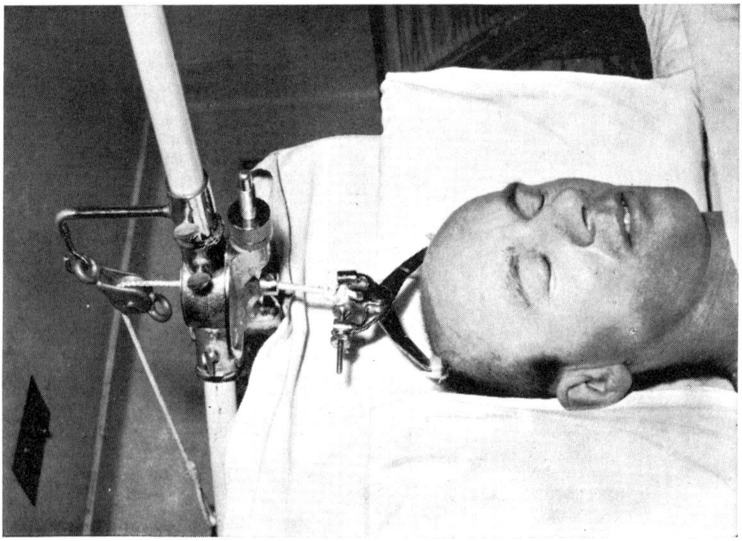

Fig. 5.8F, Skull traction, using Crutchfield calipers; the cord passes through a hole in the pivot system to which the stretchers are clamped. During turning, the line of pull remains unchanged.

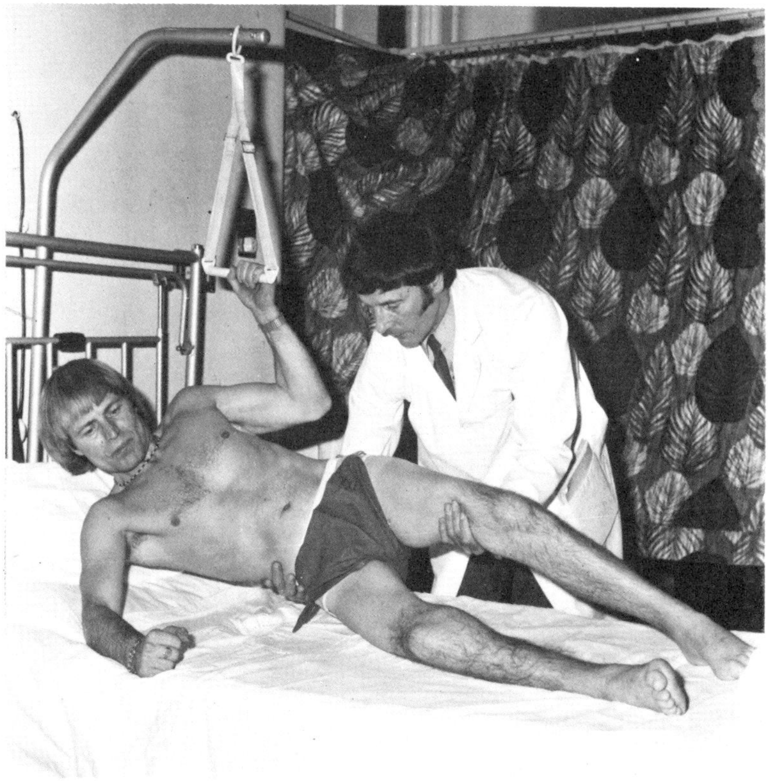

Fig. 5.9 A paraplegic patient using a monkey pole to good effect, helping his nurse. The moral-boosting effect of some independence cannot be overestimated.

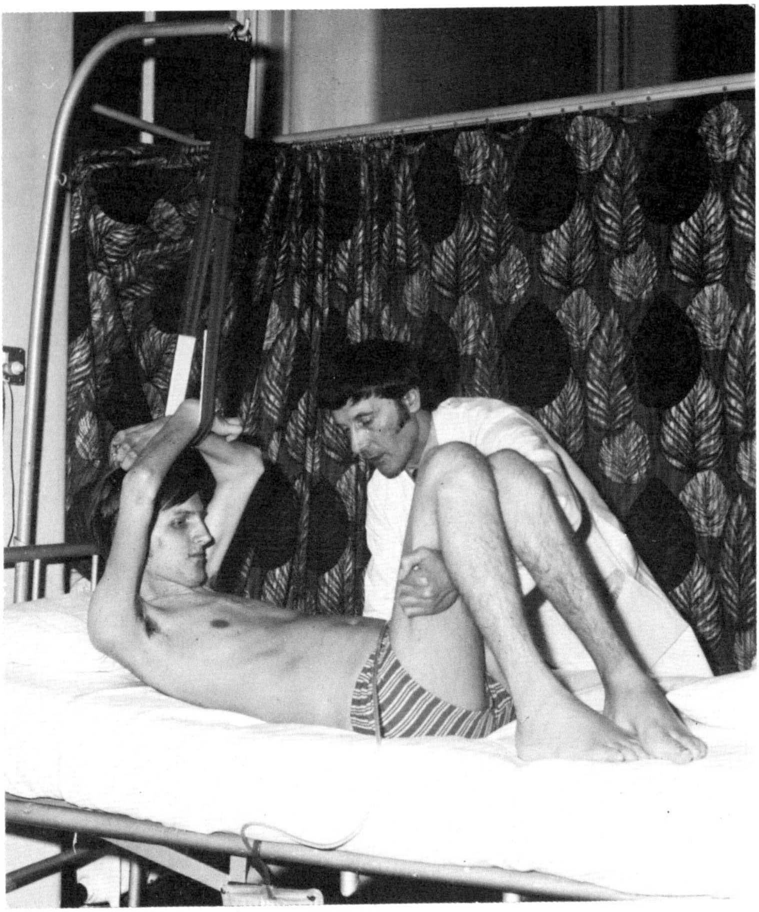

Fig. 5.10 With more care, a tetraplegic patient can assist in his turning routine. It is important to gauge how much each individual can do; if too much is asked, he will become very depressed.

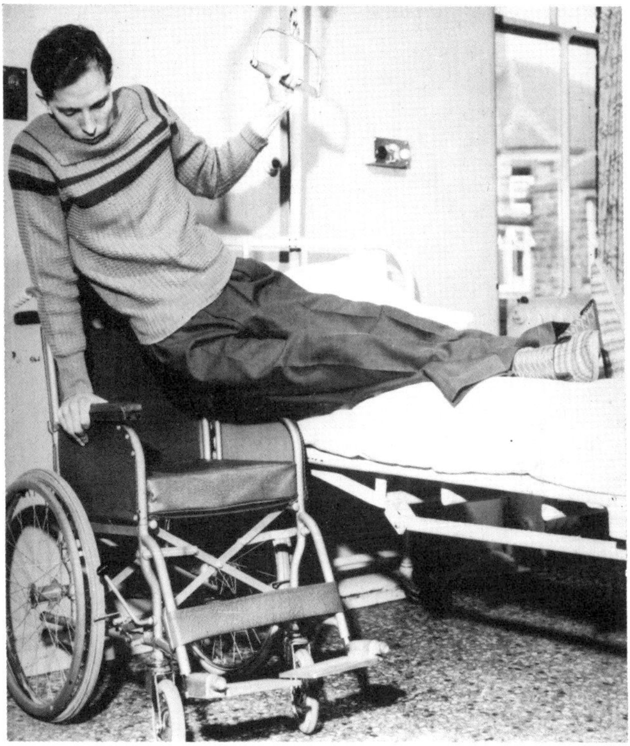

Fig. 5.11 A paraplegic patient getting from his bed into a wheelchair. All details must be taught especially the importance of ensuring that both the bed and chair wheels are locked securely.

deprived of their blood supply. At this stage, rigid attention to the avoidance of further pressure on the part can allow the inflammation to settle and ulceration of the overlying skin may be averted. More commonly, a point of no return is reached; ulceration and infection occur, and a bed sore is formed. As has been stated, sores can heal but the scarred area is forever susceptible to further breakdown because the specialised subcutaneous tissue which overlies all bony prominences is lost; instead, tough unresilient fibrous tissue is formed and the thin

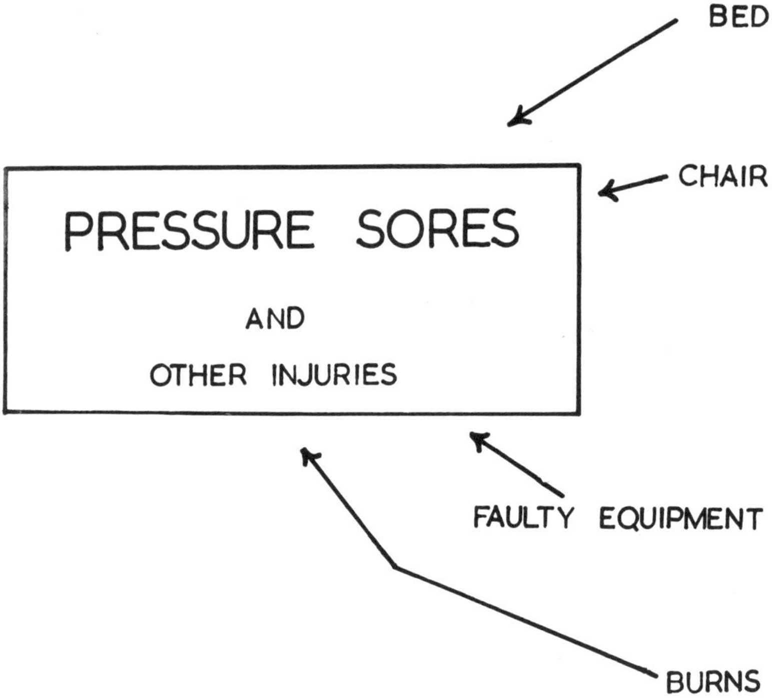

Fig. 5.12 Some causes of pressure sores and other injuries to anaesthetic skin.

overlying new skin is not cushioned, but is adherent and exposed to minor traumata (Fig. 4.1).

Healing of the ulcer can occur only after all necrotic tissue has disappeared and provided the part is shielded from further pressure. The patient is turned at frequent intervals, perhaps hourly, missing out the position in which the sore would be pressed upon. Occasionally, more than one sore has to be treated and in none of the classical positions can pressure be avoided. Great ingenuity is required in these cases and the use of large sorbo blocks judiciously spaced to avoid pressure on the ulcerated areas is valuable (Fig. 5.13).

Necrotic tissue may be allowed to separate by natural processes or

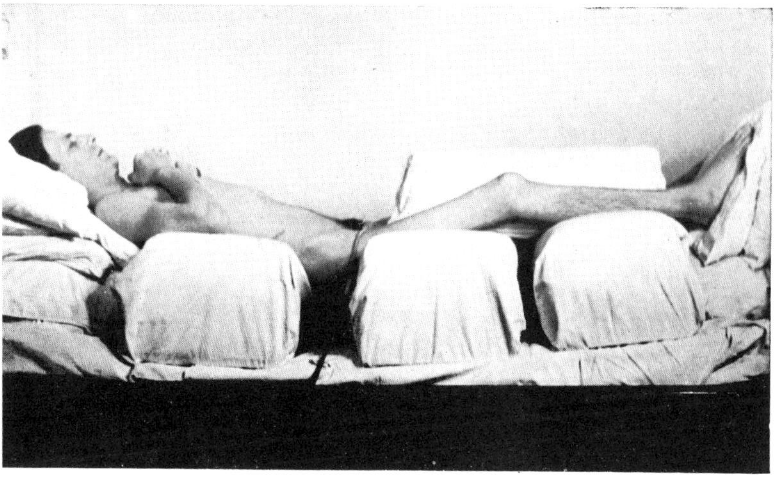

Fig. 5.13 The use of large sorbo-rubber blocks in the treatment of pressure sores. The damaged part can be suspended between the blocks and protected from further pressure.

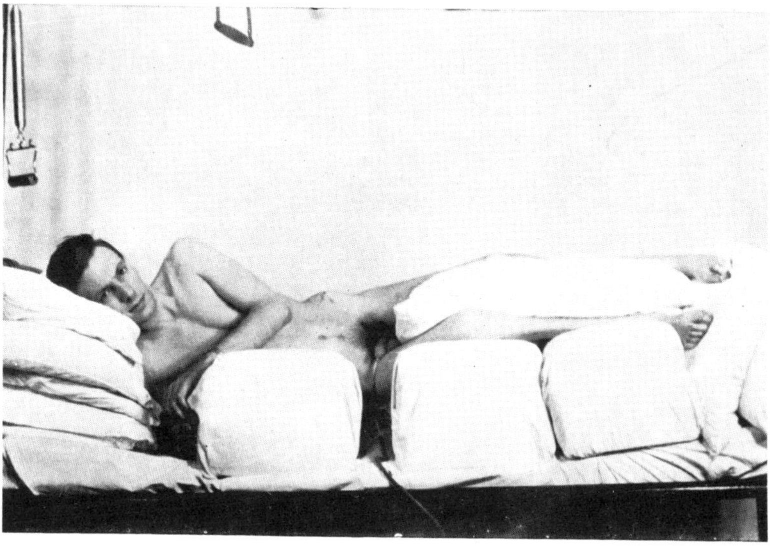

this process may be hastened, on medical advice, by surgical removal or by the application of proteolytic enzyme preparations.

Once clean, fresh granulations can grow inwards from the boundaries of the area and the cavity slowly fills. Closure is aided by contraction of the granulation tissue and completed by coverage with new skin which spreads from the surrounding skin margin; occasionally, new skin is supplied by split skin grafting. During the cleaning and granulating period, great gentleness in daily dressing should be exercised. White sterile calico is very useful because the fine weave does not entrap the young delicate granulations, as happens with ordinary

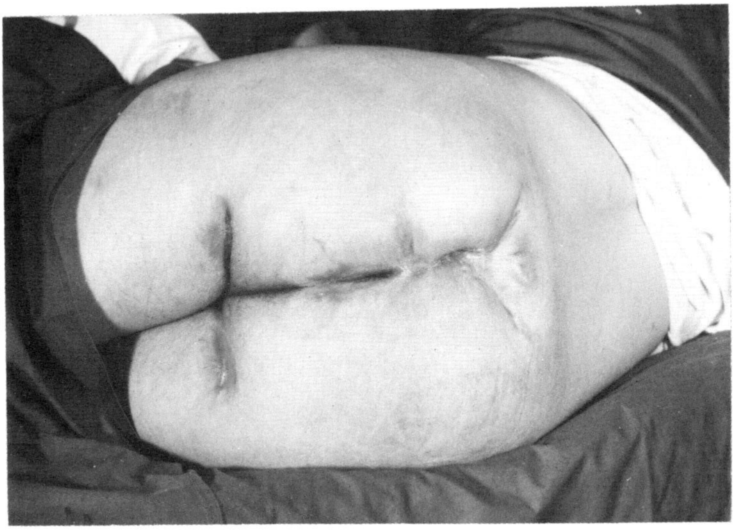

Fig. 5.14 The same sore as shown in Figure 5.1 after healing by natural processes.

gauze. The dressing should be applied dry (it will soon moisten with exudate) or, in the presence of necrotic tissue, oxidising agents such as Eusol or hydrogen peroxide help to keep the area inoffensive. In applying such agents, however, it should be borne in mind that putrifying organisms, though offensive, often aid the process of slough separation. In the later stages a simple saline dressing to prevent drying is best. Dressings should be held in place by smoothly applied flexible strapping; this should not be stretched under tension or excoriation of the skin margins is likely. When near the anus, the margins of the dressing should be lined with waterproof adhesive strapping, but the whole dressing should not be covered by this material since it encourages sogginess. A sore treated conservatively is shown in Figure 5.14.

Occasionally, plastic operations are performed to hasten healing or replace scarred unstable areas.

This description furnishes an outline of treatment, but pressure sores at different sites present varying problems of interest and importance.

1. *Sacral sores*

These can become enormous, the whole posterior aspect of the sacrum being exposed. Extension downwards can involve the perineum. The large areas heal surprisingly well although sinuses do sometimes persist, usually originating from some piece of necrotic tissue (commonly fascia or ligament, rarely bone). While open, they afford a potent loss of protein-rich fluid, therefore a careful watch should be kept on the haemoglobin level and protein intake.

In order to prevent sinus formation, pockets of dead space underlying the edges of the skin must be avoided, and if found they should be laid open. When the whole floor is covered by granulation tissue, skin cover can be aided by split skin grafting. Before grafting the surface should be swabbed and, if there is a heavy growth of pyogenic bacteria, an effort should be made to sterilise the area by the application of topical antibiotics (neomycin and bacitracin are valuable agents), and exposure to ultraviolet light or sunlight, if possible, should be arranged. These are medical considerations. Occasionally, large-scale plastic operations prove necessary for sacral sores.

2. *Ischial sores*

Ulceration over the ischial tuberosities presents special features and ulcers on the heels are similar in certain respects. Overlying the ischia is specialised weight-bearing soft tissue consisting of coarse fibrous septa which enclose large fat cells. This provides a cushion between the bony knob of the ischium and the skin; when seated on a hard surface, the subject can, as it were, roll the ischial tuberosities over different areas of skin; the areas are mostly at risk in prolonged unrelieved sitting or from badly fitted calipers. Necrosis of this tissue deprives the part of its cushion and in addition, because of the excess of fibrous tissue, these sores take months to clean and the tough slough to separate. Consequently, the healthy margins tend to scar, and the result is a tube of fibrous tissue, partly covered by skin from the surrounding margins; the ischial tuberosity, barely covered by scanty granulations, or by the ligaments normally attached to it, lies at the apex of the cavity (Fig. 5.15). This state of affairs, once established, will not heal. Less advanced examples which do heal are highly unstable and likely to break down because of the loss of the specialised weight-bearing tissue.

Surgical procedures may be necessary. The slough is excised, including the whole necrotic area, and sometimes part of the ischium (Fig. 5.16). A flap of muscle and skin may be swung across the large defect which results, and sutured primarily, or the cavity may be

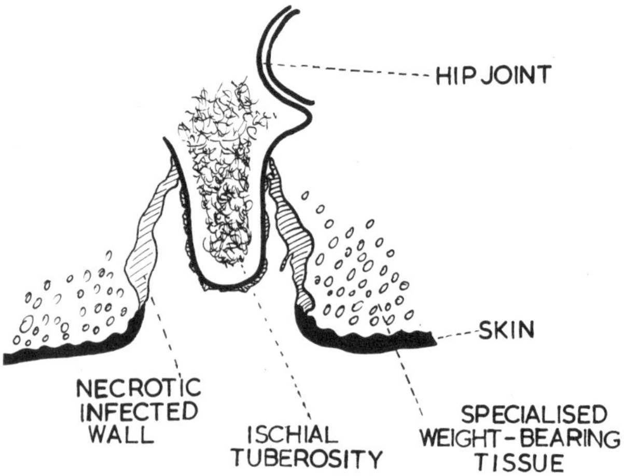

Fig. 5.15 Section of an ischial sore with bone of ischial tuberosity protruding into it; the specialised weight-bearing tissue which normally protects this bone is lost. Note the close proximity of the hip joint.

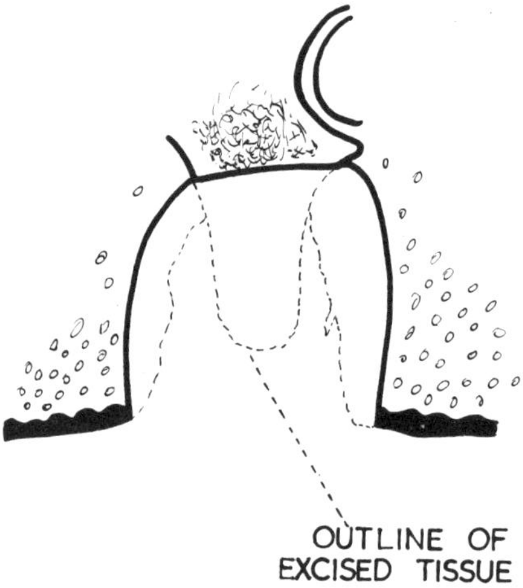

Fig. 5.16 Surgical treatment is often required for fully developed ischial sores. All dead tissue is removed, including the protruding bone.

allowed to granulate (Figs. 5.17 and 5.18). When healing by granulation (healing by second intention) is permitted, a tough adherent scar eventually forms (Fig. 5.19); the new skin is fixed and exposed to trauma from friction. It may be wise to replace the adherent scar by healthier tissue at a plastic operation similar to that shown in Figure 5.18. In cases where an unstable scar has formed, it may be advisable to plane down the knob of the ischium so that a flatter, less protuberant bont is created and the weight on the skin is distributed more evenly; the blood supply to the tissue is enhanced by this procedure.

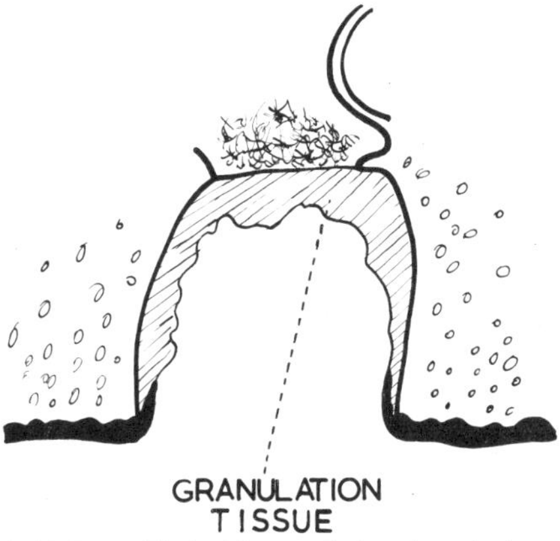

Fig. 5.17 An excised ischial sore filled with granulation tissue in the process of healing by second intention. Eventually this becomes covered by new skin which grows in from the ulcer margins.

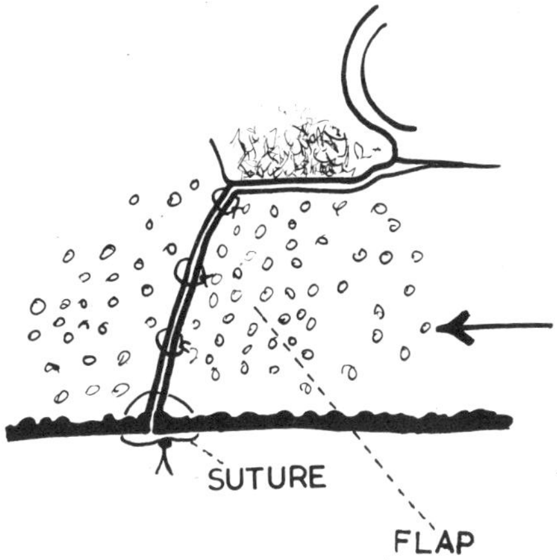

Fig. 5.18 Plastic surgical procedures are sometimes very helpful. In this diagram a flap of healthy, normal tissue has been drawn across the cavity and sutured, thus affording a better protection against further ulceration.

3. *Trochanteric sores*

Often these are the most difficult sores to persuade to heal; their formation is a tragedy. The reason for this is that, as can be seen in Figure 5.20, the skin of the trochanteric region overlies a thin muscle (tensor fascia lata) which itself is enclosed in two layers of fascia (fascia lata of the thigh). When only the skin and fat have died, healing is straightforward, but when the fascial layers are penetrated, the ulcer communicates with a large space beneath the fascia lata (Figs. 5.21 and 5.22). Further, during hip movements the ulcer margin rides forwards and backwards over the prominence of the greater trochanter. Before healing can occur, the space beneath the fascia lata must be allowed to obliterate and seal off around the ulcer margins. Chronic infection and constant movement of the hip will make this impossible. The margins of the ulcer become thickened and ring-like; abortive attempts by the skin margins to cover the constantly moving floor of the ulcer merely succeed in covering the edges of the ring alone, and ensure the impossibility of further coverage.

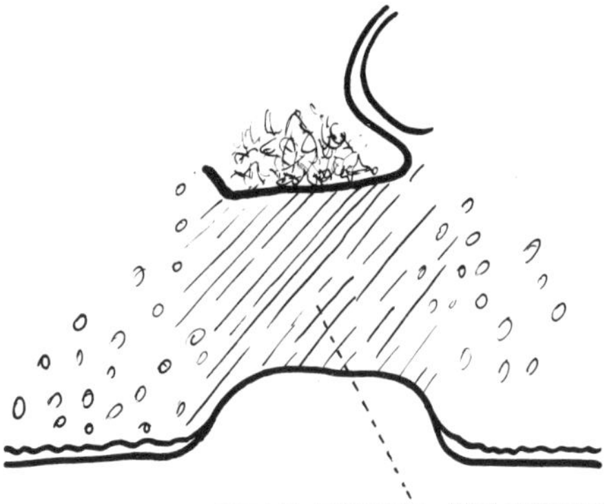

Fig. 5.19 In a sore left to heal by second intention the cavity slowly fills with granulation tissue which contracts and finally becomes covered by new thin skin; a dense adherent scar remains which is always prone to further ulceration.

Attempts at plastic procedures to swing flaps across the hole often fail because of the chronic sepsis in the subfascial plane. Healing can only be achieved by eliminating sepsis and immobilising the area. If the bone of the trochanter has been infected, the upper third of the femur may have to be resected, but when there are healthy tissues over the trochanter, this step can be avoided; especially in young people, this is most desirable, for walking is seldom possible after such an operation. The hip must be kept in full extension and not flexed; by this means the ring of the ulcer does not keep moving over the trochanter, and healing of the fascia over the vasti and gluteus medius and the under surface of the fascia lata can occur. This immobility of the hip joint can result in stiffness of the joint which may be difficult to loosen later. Skin grafting may be possible when the sealing process is complete. The healing of trochanteric sores may take many months but is worth while in young patients; in the elderly or in a high cord lesion, resection of the upper femur may be justified in that healing is expedited.

4. *Ankle, heel and foot sores*

Pressure necrosis can occur in the skin and subcutaneous tissues of the ankles and heels when in bed, and on the sole of the feet when

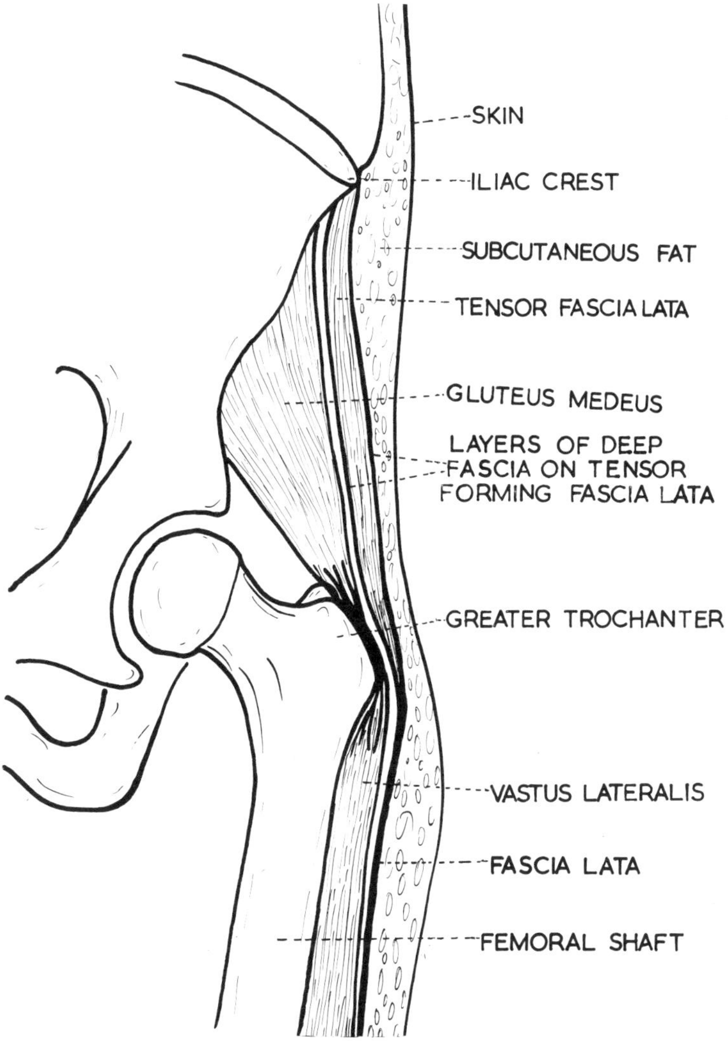

Fig. 5.20 Vertical section through the trochanteric region. The greater trochanter is seen to be superficial and protected only by skin, fat and fascia. It is evident that the trochanteric prominence is exposed to pressure risks.

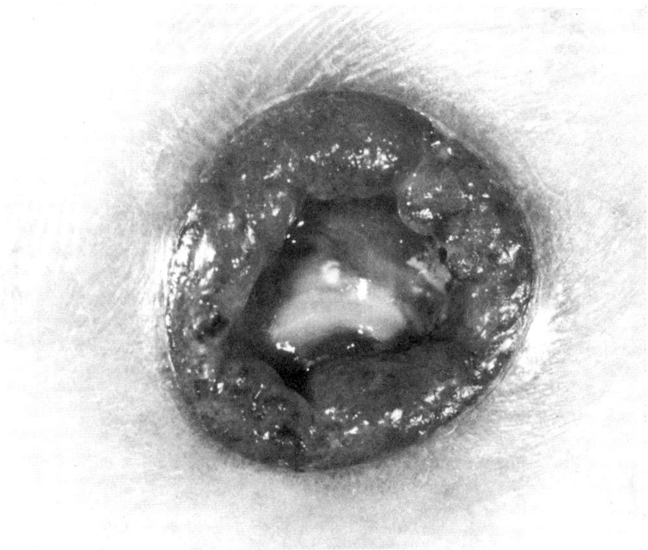

Fig. 5.21 A small but fully developed trochanteric pressure sore. It measured 3·5 cm in diameter.

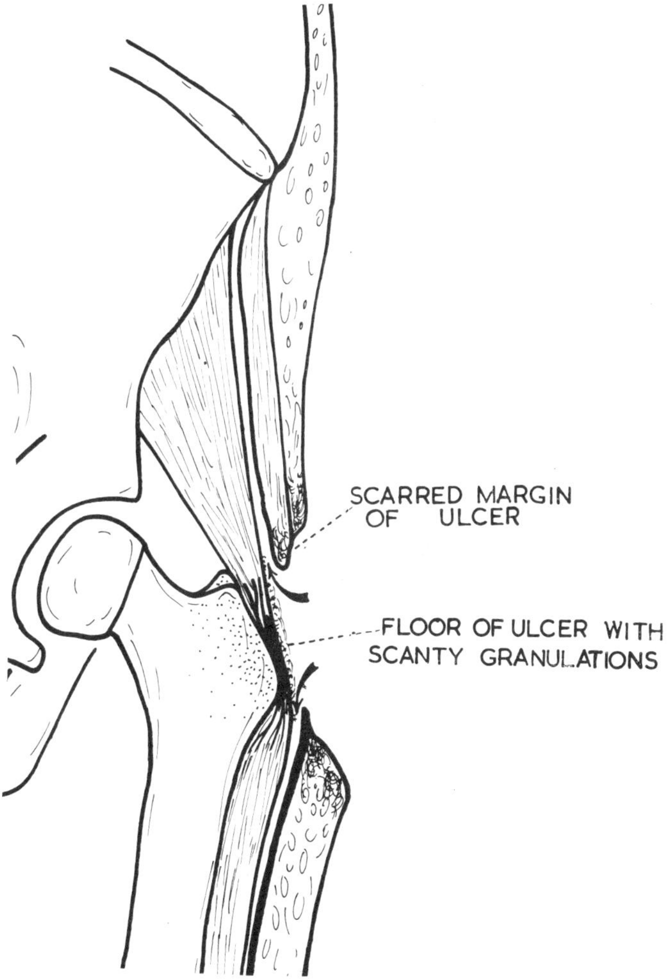

Fig. 5.22 A trochanteric sore. The arrows show the mobile plane between the fascia lata and the underlying muscle. The ring-like margin of the ulcer becomes thickened and tough, and the floor is covered by poor quality granulation tissue. The bone of the greater trochanter can become infected.

ambulant. Ulceration involves loss of the specialised weight bearing tissues, healing is slow and the scar tissue liable to further breakdown. Heel rings can be dangerous because the whole weight of the limb is born on a very small area. Fleece-lined bootees are of value occasionally.

Sores can occur anywhere but the sacral, ischial, heel, ankle and trochanteric sites are the most common. Their management is a combined medical and nursing programme. Their occurrence is a shame and can often be avoided.

6. The Prevention of Spasm

Spasm is a very difficult condition to control and treat and, although many of the aggravating factors are known, there are still gaps in our knowledge of its origin and variability. There is no single method of management and there are some types of spasm which can be controlled only by the most drastic of measures. However, spasm can be greatly minimised by paying attention to *all* the possible sources of irritating afferent stimuli which reflexly bring about the uncontrolled movements in the trunk and limbs. The commonest sources of irritation are:

1. Pressure sores
2. Urinary tract infections
3. Bladder distension
4. Bowel distension
5. Tight clothing and badly fitting appliances
6. Emotional upset (in incomplete cord lesions)
7. Joint contractures and deformities.

The first three items are discussed elsewhere.

Contractures are prevented by repeatedly manipulating all joints through their full range of movement, and *gently* stressing the limits of the range in each direction, several times a day. By this means, the capsule and adjacent soft tissues are kept supple and of normal length, and shortening, which causes contractures, does not occur. It is stressed that these passive movements are performed with the greatest gentleness; forceful stretching does much more harm than good; this applies especially in the small joints of the fingers. Obviously, the manipulations are only necessary in the paralysed parts and active exercises must be encouraged for the rest of the body. They are performed usually by a physiotherapist whose work here is of great importance (*see* Chap. 12).

Another adjunct to maintaining full ranges of movement is the careful placing of the paralysed limbs each time the patient is turned. As can be seen in the figures illustrating a turning technique, in the lateral positions the upper limb is kept fully extended at the hip and knee, while the foot is held neutral by a firm block mattress or biscuit at the foot of the bed. In the supine position the limbs are allowed to relax comfortably. If tolerated, during the later stages of treatment, the prone position has many advantages; in addition to holding the lower limbs fully extended, the stimulation of weight bearing on the front of the thighs affords benefit in increasing the reflex tone of the quadriceps. At no time, however, are the joints held rigidly at the limit of a particular movement; the capsular strain and irritation which results from this tension if prolonged is experienced, for example, when the normal individual sits with his feet on another chair and his knees, which are unsupported, sag into full extension; the backs of the knees soon ache intolerably. In the paraplegic patient this irritation could stimulate spasm, although the patient would not experience any actual pain if his cord lesion is complete.

The treatment of spasm

Sometimes cases are encountered in which, despite every care, spasm occurs, persists and is troublesome. This is seen in both complete and incomplete lesions, but is more common and often painful in incomplete cases. Painful spasm is one of the most distressing features of spinal disorders. It must be treated at its source and not symptomatically by strong analgesics or narcotic drugs; addiction is easily acquired.

The aim of treatment is to damp down the afferent limb of the reflex perpetuating the muscle contraction. Examples of methods of treatment used are mentioned below, but the choice is often difficult; some are destructive procedures.

1. *Removal of irritant foci,* notably bladder infection or distension, bowel distension, bed sores and sometimes psychological distress.

2. *Measures to strengthen the muscles which oppose those in spasm.* Passive stretching of the spastic muscle groups: as already described, if this is done by the physiotherapist several times a day during the phase of returning reflex activity, no one muscle group is allowed to become dominant. Thus if flexor spasm is minimised, reflex activity is encouraged in the extensor groups which would otherwise have become inhibited and wasted. Many patients can be taught how to perform their own passive exercises. Standing in calipers and lying prone are two excellent means of minimising flexor spasm at the hips and knees.

3. *Division of tendons and muscles (tenotomy and myotomy).* In the lower limbs the strong flexors of the hip and knee can readily be divided and at the ankle the tendo achilles can be lengthened to correct spastic plantar flexion of the feet. The selection of cases to benefit by these procedures is very much a matter of assessment of the balance of power between one muscle group and another.

4. *Division of nerves (neurotomy).* The nerve supply to some muscle groups can be selectively identified and divided. The powerful adductor muscles of the thighs are largely controlled by the obturator nerves, the division of which not only reduces the spasm in the adductor muscle group but reflexly in many other muscle groups.

Branches of the sciatic nerve can also be selected and divided.

5. *Drugs*. There are many drugs advertised as suitable for the relief of spasm. Their value and use is very much a matter of medical experience and prescription. Undoubtedly some benefits can be obtained by the careful use of drugs which depress activity at some point in the reflex arc. Care is needed to avoid side effects appearing in both the paralysed and non paralysed parts of the body.

6. *Central destructive procedures*. These attack the cause of the trouble at the level of the spinal cord. Surgical section of cord roots (rhizotomy), section of the cord itself (myelotomy) or even resection of several segments (cordectomy) are required occasionally. More commonly, reflex activity can be reduced by intrathecal injections of phenol or alcohol in varying strengths. Chemical suppression of reflex activity cannot be as selective as root section and its use is limited when it is desired to preserve useful reflexes associated with bladder and bowel activity.

7. The Prevention of Urinary Complications

Ill health and death during the later stages in spinal cord injuries are still most usually due to urinary infection and renal failure. *Persons looking after this aspect of management have the highest responsibilities.*

If the management of the bladder has been efficient during the early stages of spinal cord injury satisfactory bladder emptying can be achieved. The aims of all methods of management are the avoidance of infection, and the establishment of some form of compensatory micturition. In some patients there is intermittent and periodic voiding without sensation or control; although this may be physiologically satisfactory it is not socially safe and a portable urinal is required at all times. Other patients can initiate micturition by tapping or pressing on the lower abdomen. Still others are able to void by straining or by manual compression of the lower abdomen and even others require assistance from drugs such as Bethanecol or Carbachol. Many patients control bladder emptying by the careful timing and regulation of their fluid intake, as well as making use of abnormal types of bladder sensation which provide them with an indication of bladder fullness. It is always an advantage to have some sensation of bladder distension and even an awareness of bladder fullness can be a valuable aid to compensatory micturition. In high cord lesions bladder distension can produce headache, tingling sensations in the scalp and ears, dryness in the nose and throat and sweating on the face and scalp. These are the autonomic nervous system reactions which can serve as a warning sign of bladder fullness or impending micturition.

The most important requirement is that when the bladder is full it should be capable of emptying by whatever means is appropriate to the individual circumstances. Retention with overflow is totally unacceptable.

In the early stages after a spinal cord injury the bladder must be drained and kept free from infection. This is done either by a regime of intermittent catheterisation or by continuous drainage through an indwelling urethral catheter. Both methods require a rigidly aseptic technique. With intermittent catheterisation there is a need to restrict and regulate the fluid intake. With a continuous drainage programme there is a need for a high fluid intake of the order of 3 per 24 hours in order to diminish the deposition of phosphatic debris in the bladder and on the end of the catheter. Phosphatic debris provide a focus of infection which in turn predisposes to stone formation. An alkaline urine further predisposes to the formation of phosphatic debris and when there is this tendency the urine can be acidified by such drugs as Methionine and ammonium chloride. However, one should always remember debris and stones rarely form in the dilute urine which can be achieved by the simple expendient of maintaining a high fluid intake. This is particularly important during times of constitutional upset associated with sweating when the extra fluid lost has to be replaced before kidney excretion returns to normal.

Choice of catheter is influenced by three factors:

1. *The material of which it is made.* Red rubber is irritant to the urethral mucosa, latex rubber much less so, and some modern plastics are almost non-irritant. Soft rubber catheters of the Harris type are useful for intermittent catheterisation but should not be left indwelling. Any catheter is irritant to some extent for the urethral lining is highly sensitive to the pressure of foreign material.

2. *The size of a catheter.* The smaller the external diameter the less irritation there is to the urethra. The right size of catheter is the one which allows free drainage of urethral mucus between the side of the catheter and the wall of the urethra. This is usually 16 or 18 French gauge in most adult males. The narrowest part of the urethra may be at the external urethral meatus and this may require incision (meatotomy) before a catheter is passed.

3. *The method of retaining the catheter in the bladder,* should continuous drainage be required. The Foley catheter, which is usually made of latex rubber (plastic varieties are becoming available), is retained by a balloon inflated after insertion (Fig. 7.1). The Gibbon

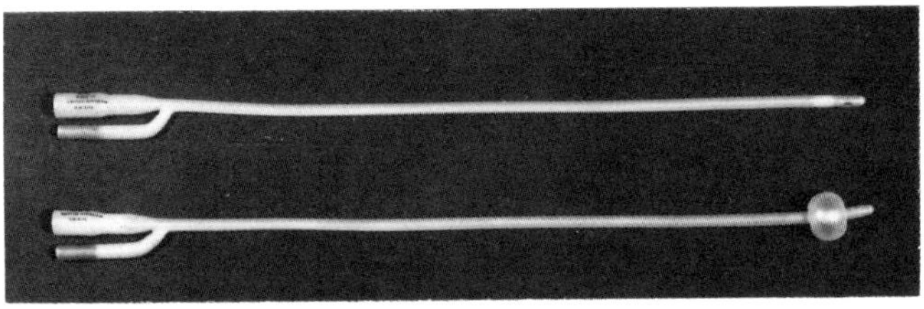

Fig. 7.1 Foley catheters, one with the ballon distended with 5 ml sterile water. The commonest sizes in use are French gauge 16–20.

catheter (Fig. 7.2) is available in very small sizes and is retained by plastic straps which have to be fixed to the skin by strapping. The Foley balloon rests continuously on the bladder neck, or worse, if the catheter tube is subjected to traction due to clumsy nursing, it can be forced down hard on to the delicate epithelium, causing irritation or even necrosis. Later, scarring is likely and automatic micturition may be prevented. On the other hand, the Foley catheter is easily retained and, provided a small size is used and the balloon only inflated with 5 ml of saline, these complications are reduced to a minimum. In the female especially, retention of the catheter other than the balloon type is not very easy, although special Gibbon catheters for the female are made.

The catheter may be introduced and, after emptying the bladder, aided by gentle suprapubic pressure, removed. Alternatively, it may be left *in situ* and changed at about weekly intervals. The choice

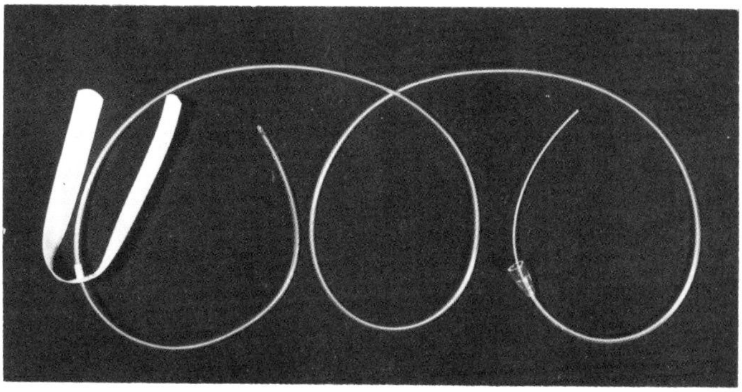

Fig. 7.2 A Gibbon catheter. Sizes range between 4 and 14 French gauge.

Fig. 7.3

A technique of catheterisation of the male patient. In this example a Foley catheter has been used and left indwelling.

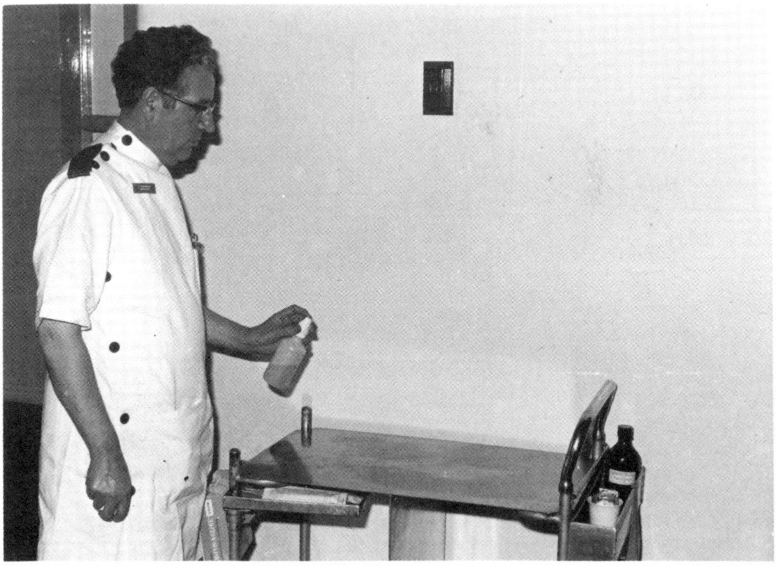

Fig. 7.3A, A stainless steel trolley is sprayed and cleaned with an aerosol antiseptic.

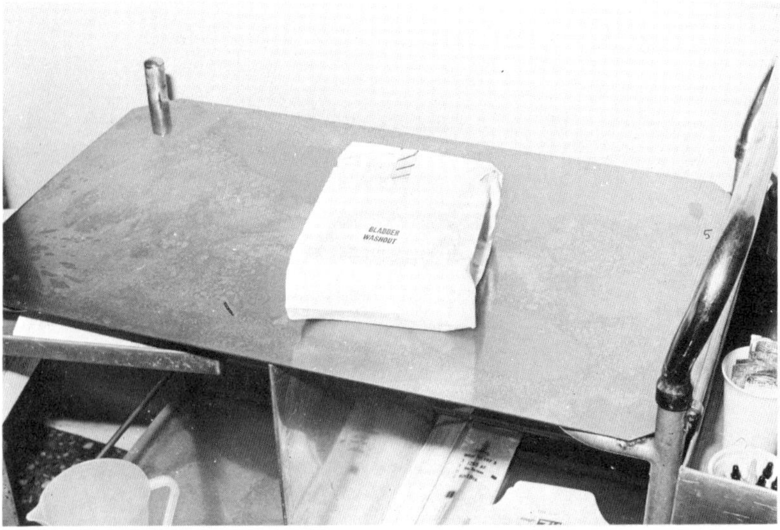

Fig. 7.3B, The bladder pack from the Central Sterile Supplies Department contains all the necessary sterile equipment.

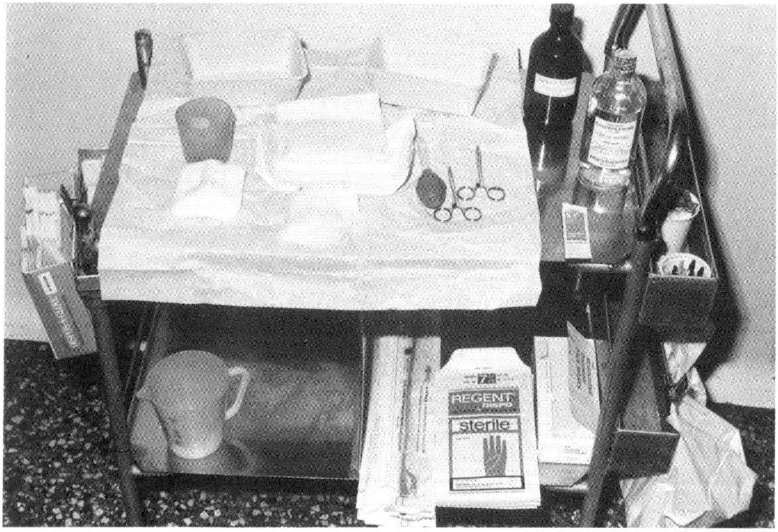

Fig. 7.3C, The trolley and pack opened out.
Top tray
On the left: sterile towels, swabs, small bowl for solutions, irrigating syringe, forceps.
On the right: antiseptic solution; bladder washout solution, sterile lubricating jelly, 10 ml syringes.
Bottom tray
Measuring receiver, selection of sterile catheters, sterile gloves, face masks, drainage bags.

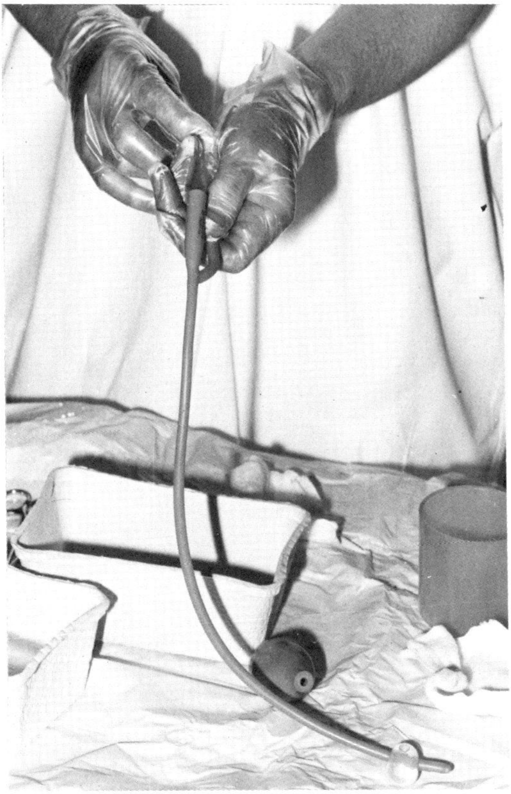

Fig. 7.3D, The Foley balloon is tested before the catheter is inserted.

between *intermittent* catheterisation or *continuous* catheter drainage is variable. Almost certainly, intermittent drainage is better; a soft rubber catheter is passed at 4- to 8-hourly intervals by a skilled person, so that the bladder is completely emptied, and between-times, regularly and moderately distended with urine as it is formed by the kidneys. It is, however, the method of choice only if a skilled technician is always available. The technician must have a clear concept of sterility and no-touch technique *and be utterly reliable;* the *slightest* abuse of sterile technique can result in infection. The same principles apply just as forcibly in passing a catheter which is to remain in the bladder.

A suitable technique of catheterisation of the male patient is described pictorially in Figures 7.3, A to M; many variations are possible, but the fundamentals of gentleness and asepsis are the same. Indwelling catheters require to be changed at weekly intervals or more frequently if the lumen is soiled.

In the female, asepsis is less easy; suitable techniques of catheterisation are described in general nursing and obstetric textbooks. An

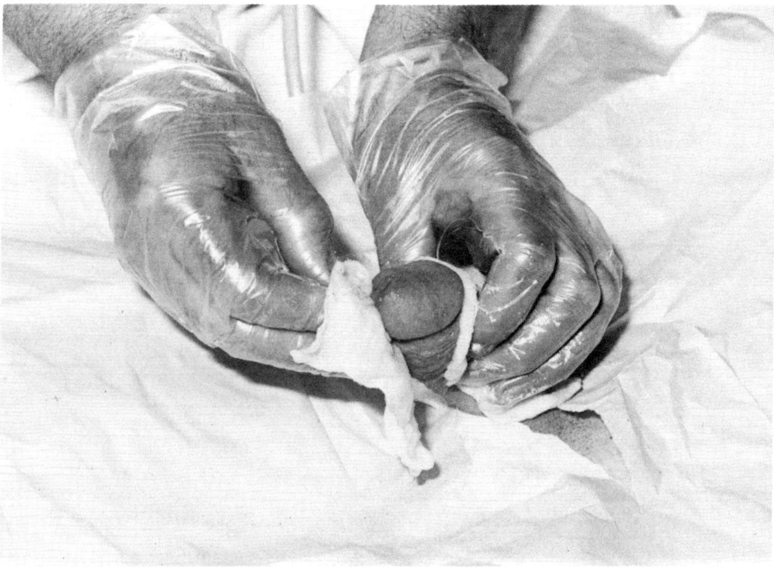

Fig. 7.3E, The penis is passed through a hole in the sterile towel and held in a dry sterile swab. The external meatus is cleaned by irrigating with sterile antiseptic solution.

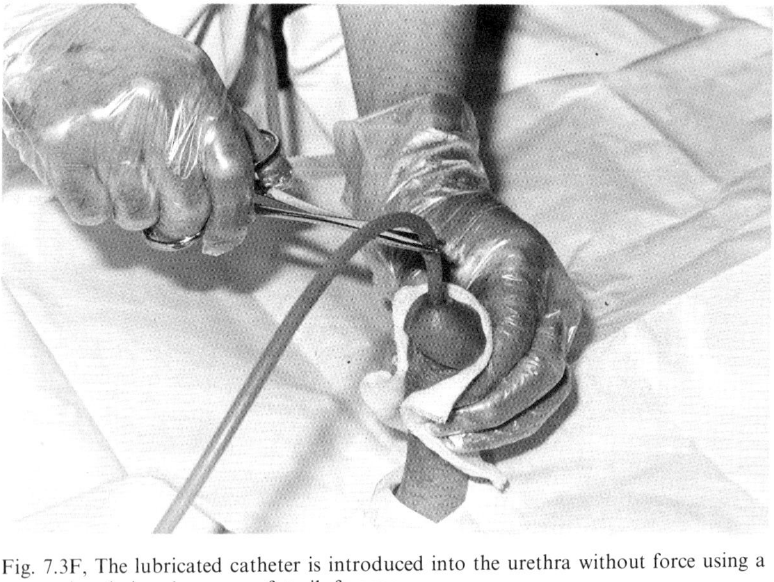

Fig. 7.3F, The lubricated catheter is introduced into the urethra without force using a no-touch technique by means of sterile forceps.

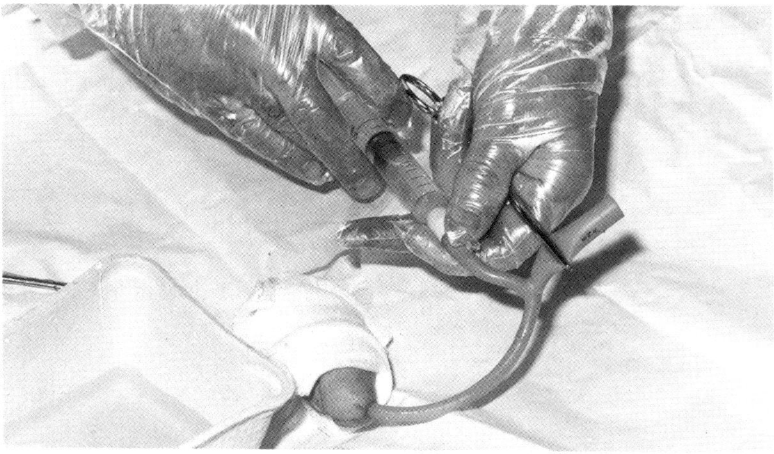

Fig. 7.3G, Once a flow of urine indicates that the tip of the catheter is well inside the bladder, the draining end is clipped-off so as to prevent the bladder from emptying completely before the balloon can be distended. If this is not done, it is possible to distend the balloon while it is still inside the urethra. Five ml of sterile water are used to distend the balloon.

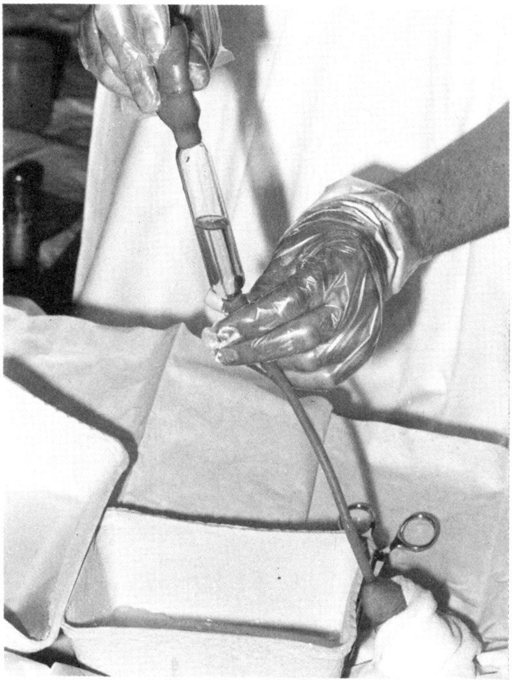

Fig. 7.3H, The catheter is now secure and the remaining urine can be drained or aspirated with the bladder syringe. If required (a medical decision) the bladder is irrigated with a selected fluid, at this stage.

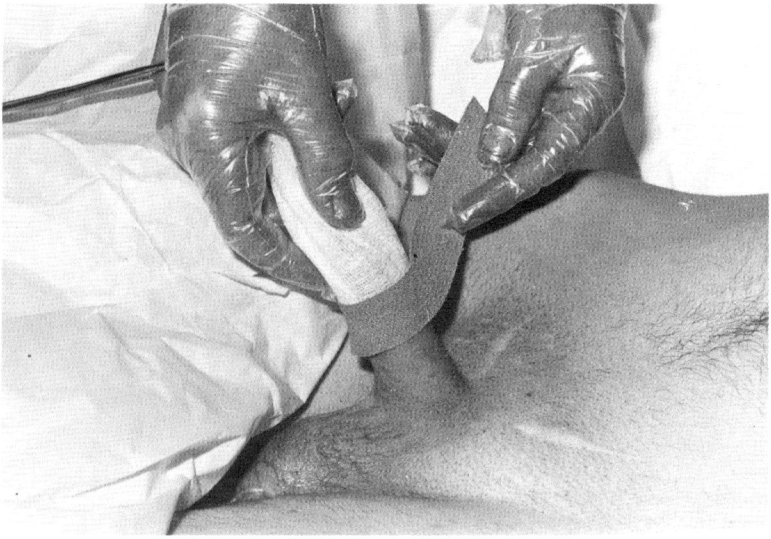

Fig. 7.3I. The end of the penis and catheter are protected with a small gauze dressing held *lightly* in position by a strip of Elastoplast; there must be no tension.

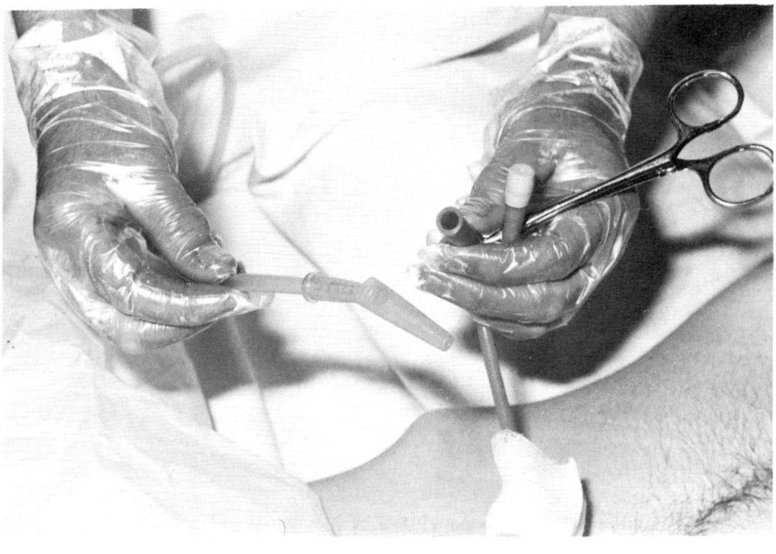

Fig. 7.3J, The end of the catheter is connected to a sterile closed drainage system.

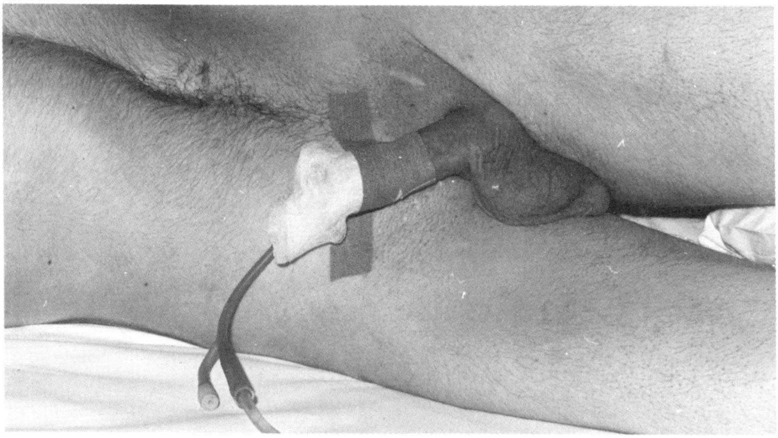

Fig. 7.3K, The penis is taped to the anterior abdominal wall with 2 cm Elastoplast. This prevents kinking of the urethra at the peno-scrotal junction. This can occur if the catheter is allowed to dangle between the patients' legs and, especially if there is tension, pressure inside the urethra can result in ulceration or even fistula formation.

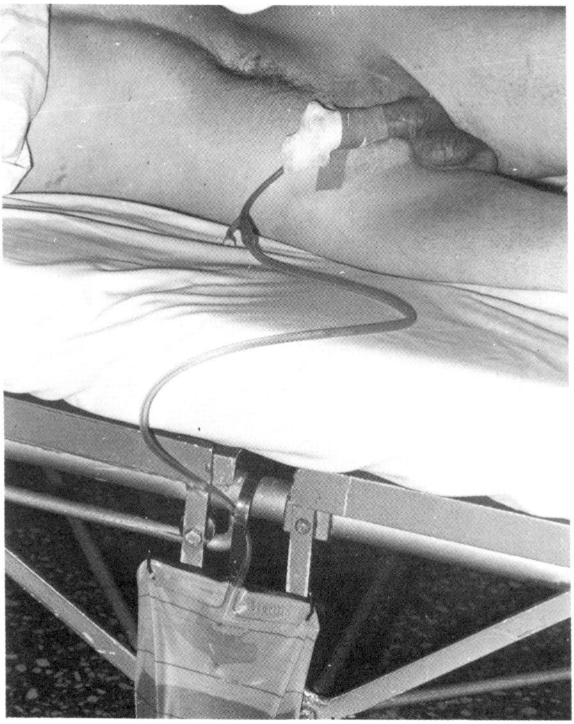

Fig. 7.3L, The completed closed drainage system using a Foley catheter and hanging bed bag; there must be no tension on the catheter or drainage tube. It is advisable to anchor the tube to the bed clothes by a safety pin positioned well away from the patient.

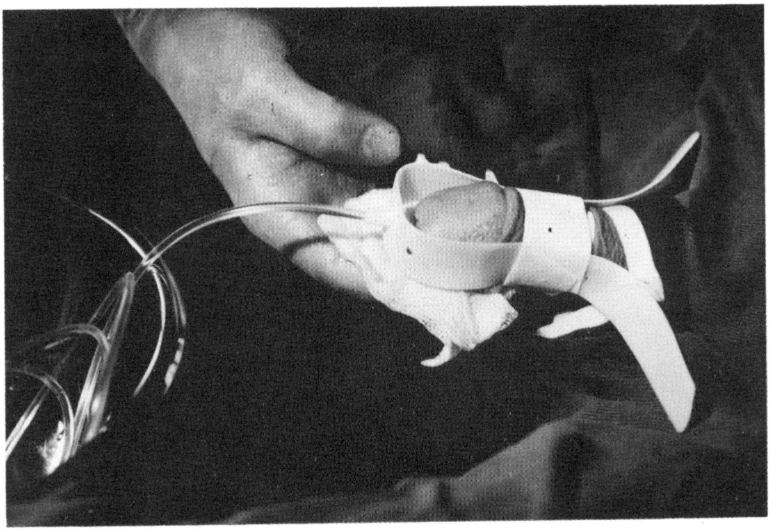

Fig. 7.3M, Shows a Gibbon catheter which has been introduced in a similar manner to the Foley catheter and secured by its plastic straps; these are retained by a *loosely* applied turn of adhesive strapping.

essential feature is that one hand of the operator is kept solely for holding separate the labia while the other cleanses the introitus and introduces the catheter; thus the one hand manipulating the catheter is kept absolutely dry and sterile. The introitus is cleansed with Savlon on swabs held by forceps. Indwelling catheters become soiled very easily and ascending infection is almost inevitable.

Both intermittent catheterisation and continuous drainage may be employed in the same centre; in others, there may be a strong preference for one or the other. It is essential that whichever method is used, it should be conducted properly.

It cannot be stressed too strongly that the operator must know how much force to use in the passing of the catheter; the normal 'feel' of the urethra is learned by experience and such experience must be acquired under the surveillance of an expert. Any alteration in the normal sensation of passing the catheter is an indication for seeking medical advice; it is so easy for the delicate urethral mucosa to be damaged by forceful passage of instruments or catheters. It is no loss of pride to be unable to pass a catheter; on the contrary, it is a token of skill to appreciate abnormal resistance. In the event of abnormal resistance, a catheter is not the right instrument for investigating its cause. Steel introducers or bougies are never within the province of the nursing or technical staff.

Catheterisation should be performed in a special room; sometimes it is said that the urine of a patient on catheter drainage cannot be kept sterile—this is simply not true; both intermittent and continuous drainage systems *can* maintain the urinary tract free from infection if established meticulously.

Towards the end of the period of spinal shock the bladder will begin to show evidence of reflex activity on filling. If the method of

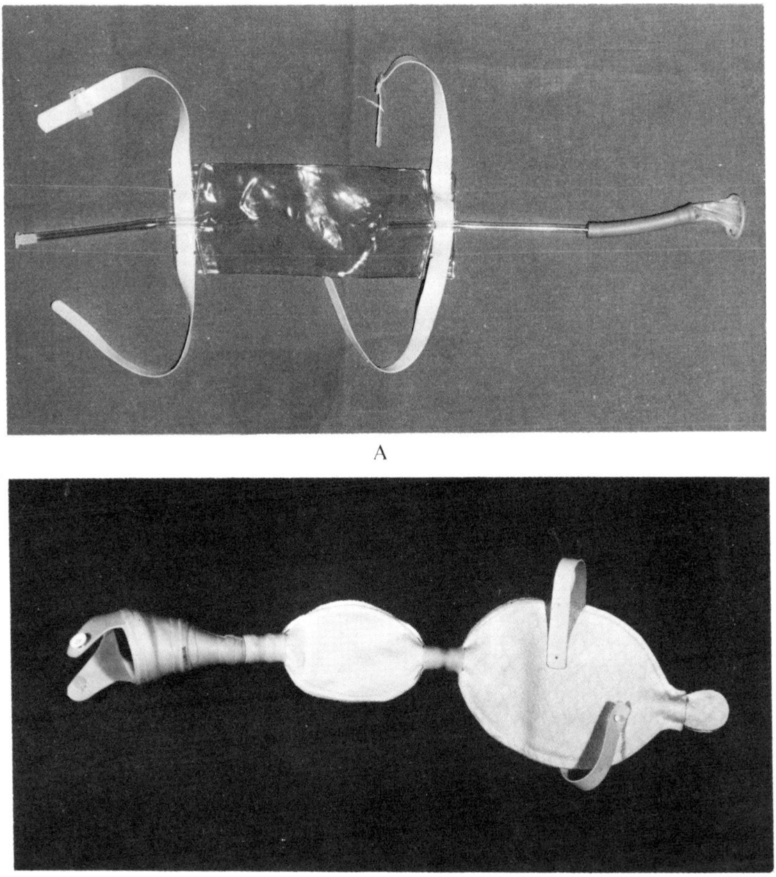

A

B

Fig. 7.4 Male urinal appliances. A, A condom urinal with connecting tube attached to a polythene collecting bag and retaining straps. B, Composite sheath type urinal with double leg bags and retaining straps.

intermittent catheterisation is being used the patient may have spontaneous voiding of small amounts of urine in the intervals between the catheterisations. If the continuous method is in progress it may be noted that urine is voided down the side of the catheter. In the latter instance, this is the occasion for a trial period of intermittent catheterisation and the use of all measures to encourage further urine voiding whether by straining, tapping or with the help of drugs.

Care must be taken to see that the bladder does not over-distend and it may be necessary to carry out intermittent catheterisation during the day, but continue with an indwelling catheter during the night. In some centres cystometry (measurement of the pressure changes within the bladder as it fills) is used as an index of bladder activity.

Efficient micturition can be established in most cases but perfect control throughout the day and night is achieved by only a few. In the male patient, odourless collection of the urine into a urinal worn under the trousers is satisfactory. It is more convenient for men wearing a urinal if the inner seam of the trouser leg is replaced by a long zip fastener so that the bag can be emptied easily (Fig. 12.11). Two varieties of the appliance are shown in Figure 7.4. The most commonly used system for the male employs a condom connected to a plastic collecting bag. The components are assembled by the patient himself as shown in Figure 7.5. The patient must be instructed in cleaning and emptying the appliance and in inspecting the skin of the penis for sogginess and sores; these may be cured by a barrier cream or, if necessary, a period using a simple male urinal bottle. Most patients sleep at night with a bottle carefully positioned to avoid bed wetting, for involuntary micturition continues throughout the 24 hours as in a baby. Reflex micturition can be provoked in some by pressing over the bladder, stroking or tapping the lower abdomen, pinching the upper thighs or penis; each case is individual in these respects.

Sometimes, automatic micturition does not occur or is incomplete because, owing to loss of normal nervous control, the urethral sphincter does not relax adequately when the bladder contracts. The result is that emptying is incomplete and both infection and back pressure effects on the kidney contribute to early renal failure.

In these circumstances an operation is necessary to weaken the urethral sphincter. The common procedures are transurethral resection (in which an instrument is passed along the urethra and the tissue of the bladder neck divided) and pudendal neurectomy (in which the nerves supplying the sphincter are severed).

It should be noted that suprapubic cystostomy (drainage by a tube passed directly into the bladder through an incision made in the anterior abdominal wall) is rarely performed today and is not considered in this account.

Urinary management in the female

The establishment of satisfactory micturition in the female patient is very difficult because inopportune incontinence cannot be managed by an external appliance. Incontinence pads and rubber or plastic pants cause soreness and infection. More and more female patients are now being managed with bladder drainage by indwelling urethral

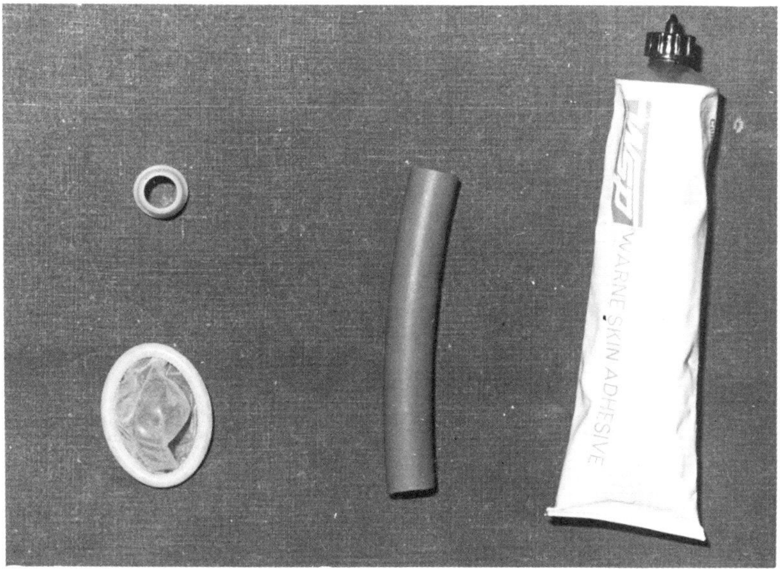

Fig. 7.5A, Component parts of the male condom urinal: condom, adaptor rubber connecting tube and adhesive cement.

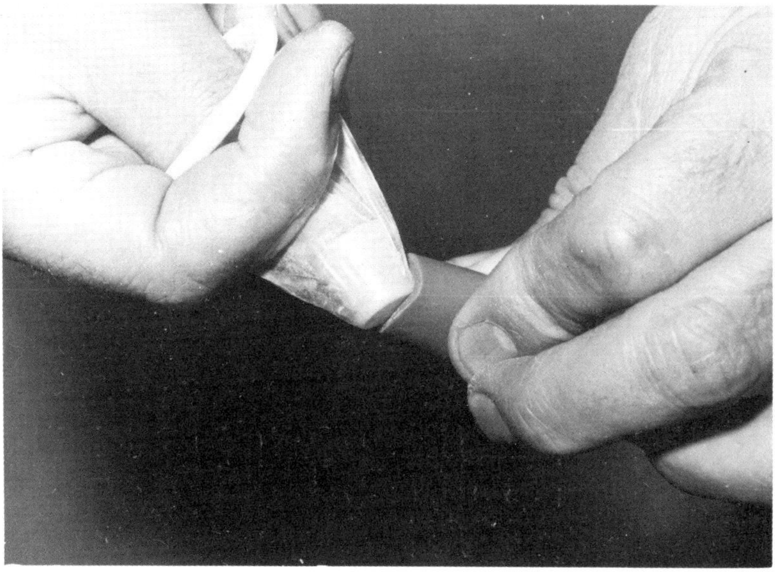

Fig. 7.5B, Condom with adaptor in place being inserted into the connecting tube.

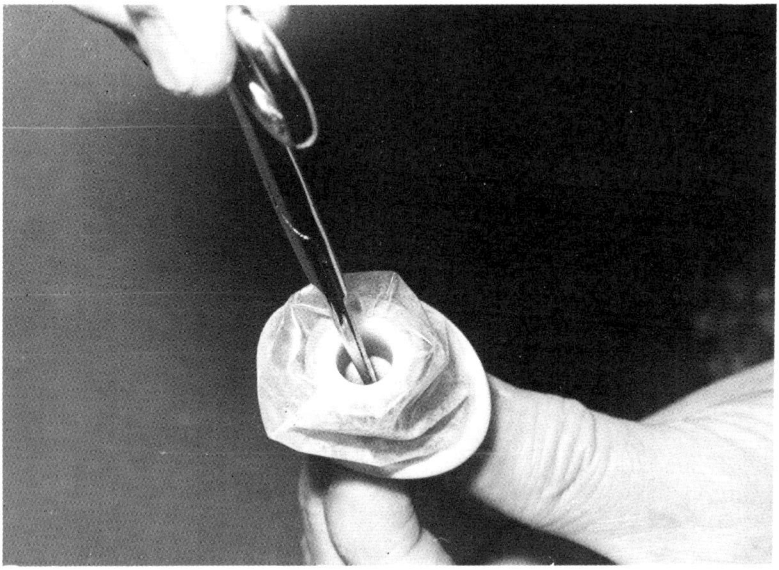

Fig. 7.5C, Condom being punctured with scissors or forceps. Note that this is not a sterile procedure.

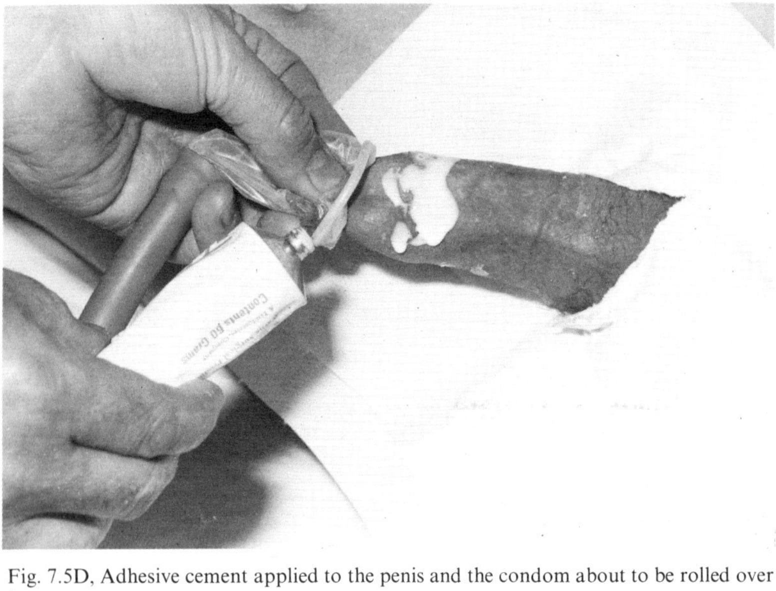

Fig. 7.5D, Adhesive cement applied to the penis and the condom about to be rolled over it.

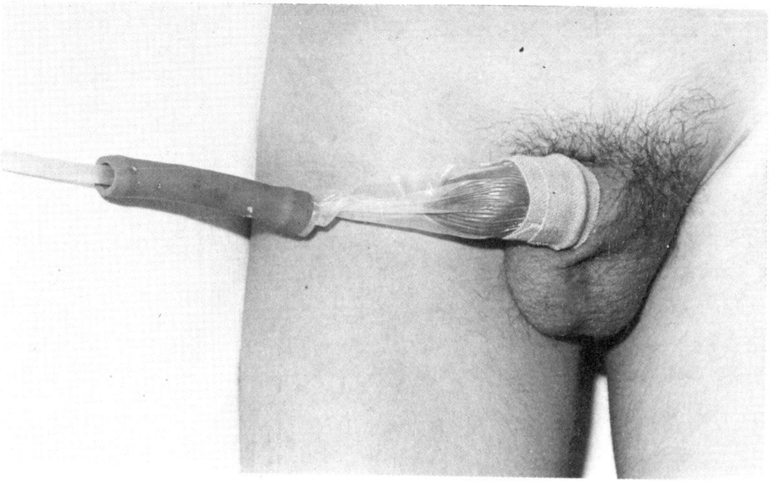

Fig. 7.5E, If necessary the adhesive can be reinforced with a turn of lightly applied elastoplast strapping.

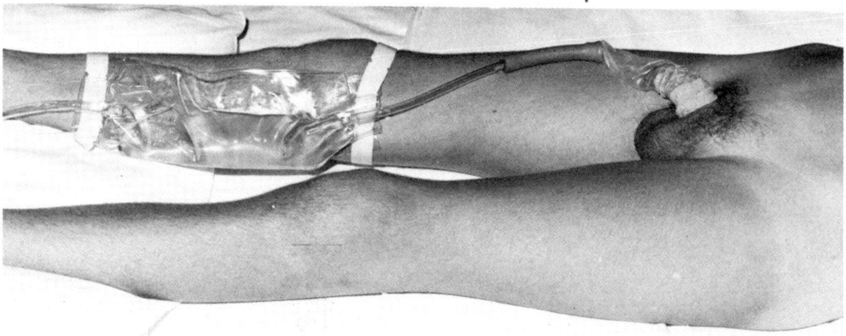

Fig. 7.5F, The assembled condom and drainage system.

catheters which can be clipped and released at regular intervals. These catheters, of course, require to be changed at regular intervals and there is a need to control infections with constitutional upset. A few patients have produced problems in the long term when bladders have contracted and the urethra become patulous. When this has occurred there has been a need to exhort to a diversion of the urinary tract by a variety of means. The commonest of these is with the use of a piece of ileum to form a conduit between the ureters and an opening on the lower abdomen (Figs. 7.6 to 7.11). Here, the urine collects and is discharged passively into a disposable plastic bag which adheres satisfactorily to the skin around the outlet of the ileal

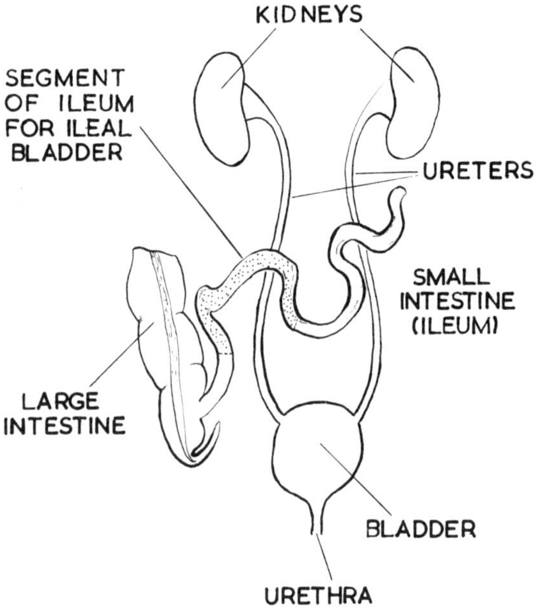

Fig. 7.6 Normal urinary drainage. The shaded portion of ileum is to be used for the construction of an ileal loop bladder.

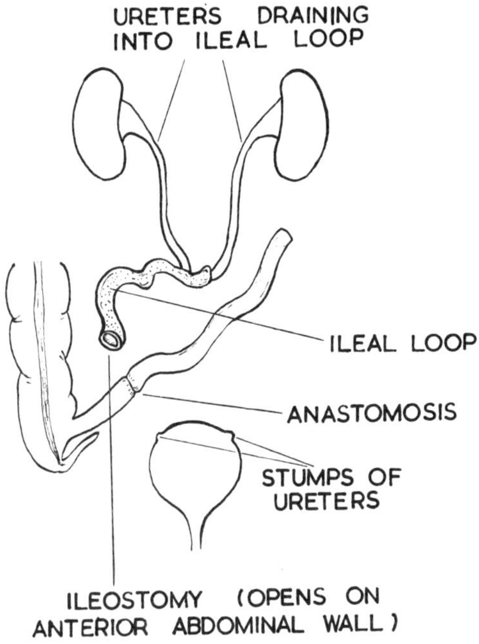

Fig. 7.7 Diversion of the urine into an ileal loop bladder.

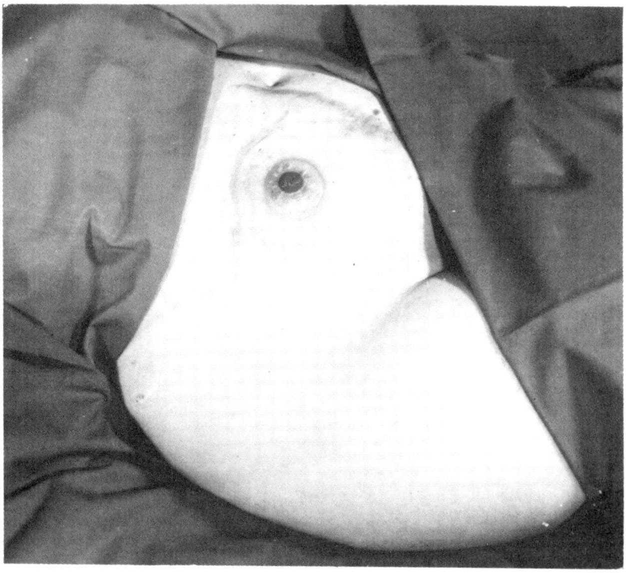

Fig. 7.8 An ileostomy.

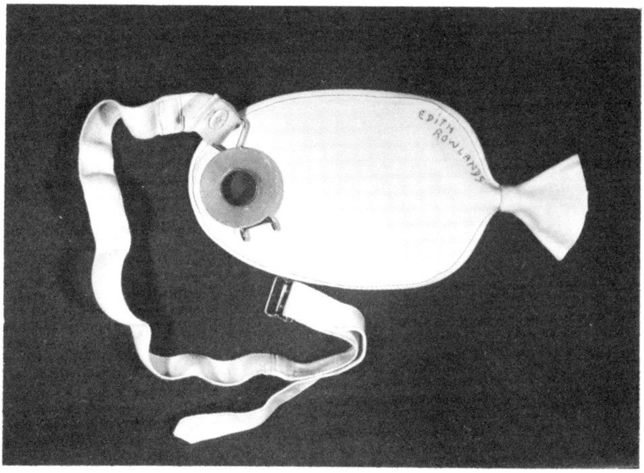

Fig. 7.9 Ileostomy bag for ileal loop bladder showing the flange which is fixed to the skin of the abdominal wall by adhesive solution.

loop or into a rubber washable bag which attaches to a plastic ring stuck to the skin around the ileostomy (Figs. 7.9, 7.10 and 7.11).

This is a major operation but many patients have been most grateful for such a solution to their problem. Other artificial methods of urinary drainage have been tried, but the ileal loop seems to be the best.

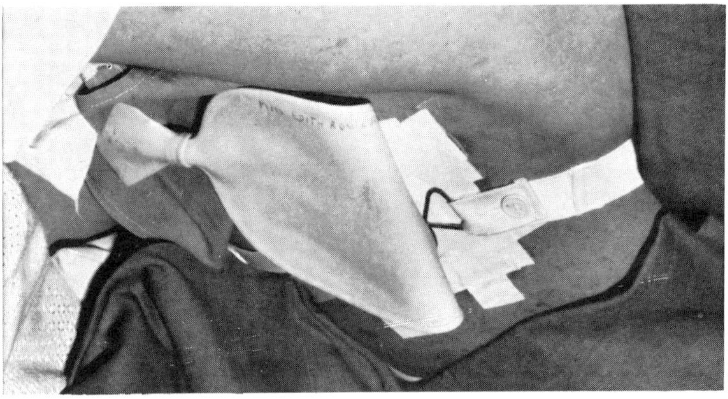

Fig. 7.10 Ileostomy bag in position.

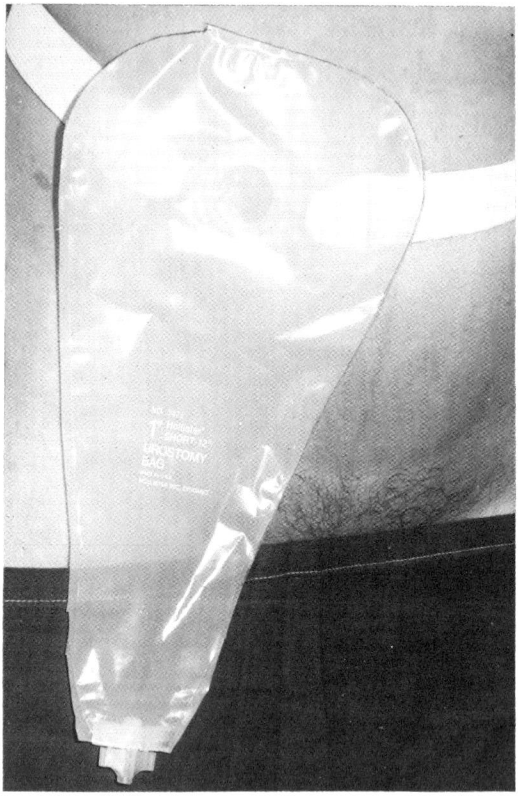

A

Fig. 7.11 A–C Polythene and skin adhesive ileostomy bag. Disposable type which is easy to apply and drain. It is changed daily.

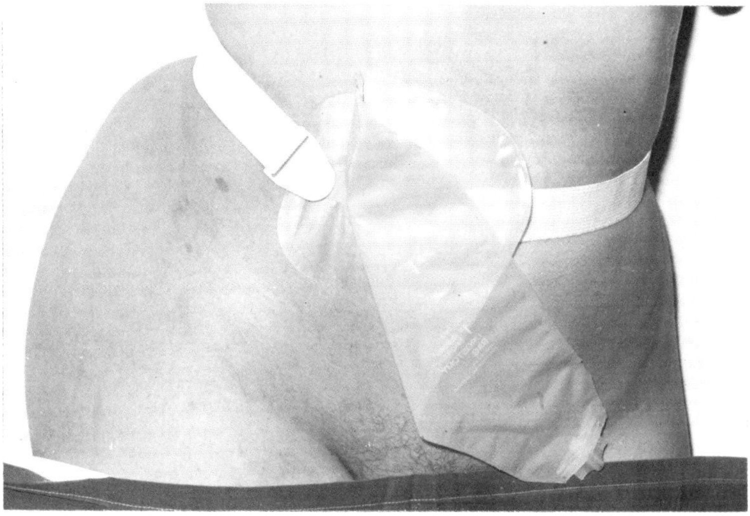

Fig. 7.11B

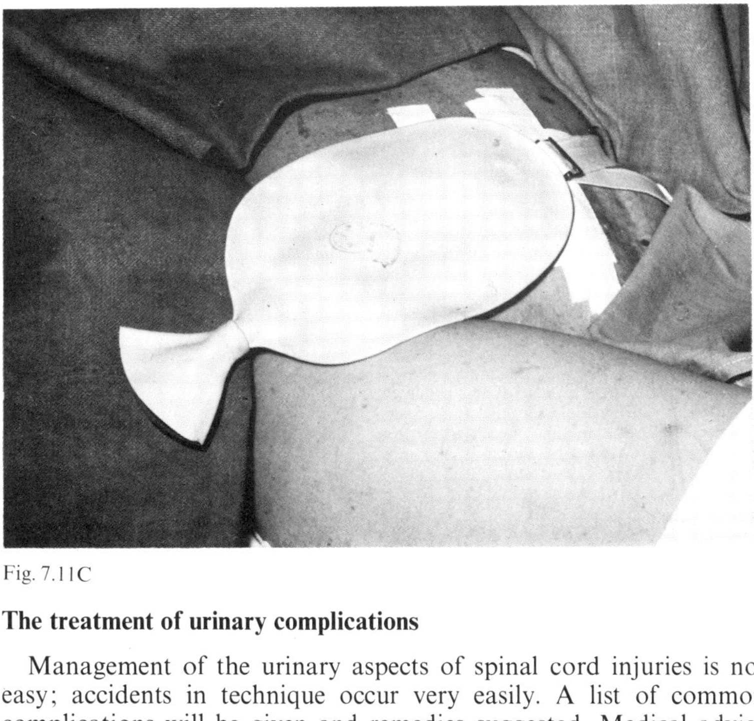

Fig. 7.11C

The treatment of urinary complications

Management of the urinary aspects of spinal cord injuries is not easy; accidents in technique occur very easily. A list of common complications will be given and remedies suggested. Medical advice is essential.

1. *Priapism*

Any stimulation of the public region or genitalia in the paraplegic male may cause an erection to occur, over which he has no control. It is not a phenomenon of sexual emotion but is purely reflex. It may be another source of severe embarrassment, and should be ignored. If the patient, in his confusion, draws attention to the situation, it is up to the nurse to treat the matter lightly, and explain it as a common happening. Priapism can be a nuisance in displacing a catheter of the Gibbon type, or can make the fitting of a urinal difficult. Any strapping around the penis should be very loose and elastic for, should an erection occur after its application, intense engorgement of the tissues may occur.

Similarly, if the prepuce (foreskin) is not pulled back into position after catheterisation, swelling can result with paraphimosis (the foreskin cannot be pulled back over the glans). In patients with a tight prepuce, circumcision may be advisable.

2. *The blocked indwelling catheter*

First, it is necessary to ascertain the cause of the blockage, e.g., the catheter may have slipped, or, in the case of the Gibbon catheter, blood, pus, or solid precipitate may have blocked the lumen. It has been mentioned already that an indwelling catheter should be changed at weekly intervals. This is because, even if kept dilute, deposits of amorphous or crystalline material on its wall can obstruct the lumen quite suddenly. In the bladder gelatinous material can collect, especially in the event of cystitis, in the form of a mixture of pyelonephritis has occurred, casts may accumulate in the bladder in large amounts.

The catheter must be removed and replaced by a moderately sized soft rubber catheter (about 14°F) and the bladder irrigated and aspirated gently and repeatedly with 0·5 per cent acetic acid or normal saline warmed to 37° to 38°C, until a clear return is yielded; a volume of about 200 to 300 ml is used for each irrigation with a Cany Ryal syringe of suitable size. After adequate irrigation, choice of further management is a medical problem. Perhaps the bladder and urethra should be left empty and regular intermittent catheterisation, with irrigation as necessary, should be instituted. If a catheter must be left in, it will have to be of moderate size, or further blockage is likely. This may be preferable only in the presence of depressed urinary function when back pressure on the kidneys must be prevented at all costs.

The nature of the obstructing agent should exercise influence in further treatment; if pus is present, the urine is infected. Blood may be due to infection, rough catheterisation or ulceration at the bladder neck from catheter pressure. (Bleeding may occur following a failed, so-called 'catheter trial' in which, after a lengthy period of continuous drainage, the catheter is simply removed and the bladder allowed to over-distend.) When solid precipitate has caused a block, the reaction of the urine should be ascertained with litmus paper and, if possible, the nature of the solid analysed in the laboratory; by changing the reaction of the urine, precipitation may cease (*see* above).

3. *Urinary infection*

Acute infection of the urine is usually manifest by a sudden pyrexia, shivering, sweating, vomiting and malaise. On culture of a catheter specimen of urine, the nature of the infecting organism can be identified, and appropriate antibiotics prescribed.

It is the nurse's duty to ensure that the patient has an adequate fluid intake of about 3 litres per 24 hours. This may have to be augmented if the patient is sweating freely and may be impossible if he is nauseated or vomiting. In these circumstances an intravenous infusion may be necessary; obviously a low fluid intake would result in concentrated urine, precipitation of solids and perpetuation of the infection. The treatment of urinary infection is in the medical province. It is to be regarded very seriously and its cause must be sought and rectified.

4. *Stone formation*

Small stones may pass naturally but larger ones in the bladder or kidney require surgical removal. They result from infection or concentration of the urine. In particular, the calcium content of the urine plays a big part in their formation and if this can be kept down, stone formation is less common. There is evidence to suggest that exercise, in particular weight bearing, helps to prevent calcium loss from the skeleton; at all times the patient should be encouraged to be as active as possible. Stones may be visible on X-ray of the abdomen or demonstrated by special X-rays of the kidneys and ureters (pyelograms); these investigations are done routinely throughout the patient's life.

5. *Epididymo-orchitis*

This condition has been explained in Chapter 3; the male genital organs are closely connected with the urinary tract at the prostate and along the vas deferens to the epididymis and testicle.

Nursing treatment consists of supporting the weight of the swollen heavy scrotum on a pidded strip of elastic strapping across the thighs. The parts should be kept clean and dry. Manual removal of faeces should be done very carefully, especially if the prostate is swollen when palpated per rectum. The patient may feel extremely ill although the severe pain normally experienced is not perceived in complete cord lesions. Antibiotics are prescribed, and, if vomiting occurs, intravenous administration of fluid is required. Abscesses form sometimes and may require surgical drainage.

6. *Failure to establish compensatory micturition*

Effective micturition may be delayed in its onset, or fail to be achieved in spite of all efforts at bladder training. The main cause of failure is neurological imbalance between bladder contraction and sphincter relaxation and the main aggravating factors are infection and subsequent scarring of the bladder wall and bladder neck. Any illness affecting the paraplegic patient in later life can alter the pattern of his micturition. Reflex activity may become less efficient or voiding by straining inadequate to produce bladder emptying. There is a tendency for an insidious increase of volume of residual urine and the occurrence of increased back pressure on the upper urinary tract. It is for these reasons that patients must be reviewed at regular intervals so that the quality and quantity of their residual urine can be measured and X-ray examinations made of the upper urinary tract. At the same time blood chemistry can be estimated. The ratio of the volume of urine voided to the volume of residual urine is probably more important than the actual volume of residual urine itself.

7. *Renal failure*

This is one of the most serious things which can happen to the patient. Frequently it is irreversible for, despite treatment, a chronic infective process continues within the kidney substance, which antibiotics cannot cure. However, another type of renal failure occurs which can be treated successfully. In this, back pressure from retention with overflow depresses renal function, and recovery after proper treatment is possible. This reversible failure is due purely to the mechanical effects of back pressure and not to irreversible pyelonephritis, although sooner or later infection is inevitable.

In either case, treatment is urgent. The back pressure is relieved by catheter drainage, infection treated, and haemoglobin level restored if necessary by blood transfusion. The whole bladder retraining programme must be repeated once satisfactory renal function has been restored. Good early management and follow-up should prevent the occurrence of renal failure.

8. The Prevention of Cachexia

The prevention of cachexia in spinal cord injuries rests largely in avoiding the complications detailed in other chapters, viz.:

Prevention of sores
Prevention of spasm
Prevention of urinary infection.

Other features of importance are:

1. Diet

Especially in tetraplegia, the appetite is often small and yet a good quality diet with moderate calorie content (2000 Calories/day) is essential. The hand-feeding of tetraplegic patients makes heavy demands on nursing personnel but it must be done assiduously. Patience and a willingness to chat between mouthfuls must balance a kind firmness in persuading the patient to eat adequate amounts of food. Often patients can help each other in this respect and should be encouraged to do so.

2. Fluid intake

This should be charted as a routine discipline. Three litres per day is a lot to drink and sometimes this is responsible for reducing the appetite. Accordingly, drinking should be largely between meals and not just before. Evening and early morning drinks can spread the load. Even when catheter-free and apparently stable as far as micturition is concerned, a fluid intake of 3 litres per day should become a routine. It is a great help if cups, mugs and beakers are of a standard size, so that for practical purposes, simple recording of fluid volumes is well within the capability of the average patient. When, of course, some complication is in process, accurate recording is essential and this must be performed by the nurse.

3. Iron supplement, and blood transfusion

These are sometimes necessary to maintain the haemoglobin concentration normal.

4. Rest

There are so many procedures in the daily routine of paraplegic and tetraplegic patients that it is easy for them to be constantly undergoing some attention, with the result that they get inadequate rest. Rest is important during the first few weeks, not only of body, but of mind, the latter being subject to considerable stress. Nursing and other procedures should not be staggered but performed in carefully balanced blocks at one- to two-hourly periods. Much will depend on the individual patient as to how much activity can be sustained without fatigue.

5. Weight considerations

It is undesirable that paraplegic or tetraplegic patients should become overweight; walking or any changing of position in bed or a chair is made much more strenuous and also, nursing procedures are more difficult. On the other hand, spare individuals with a paucity of subcutaneous tissues are more prone to pressure sores. In the presence of adequate dietary protein an excess of carbohydrate and fat is undesirable. A rigorously enforced diet must be inflicted only after consideration, and with agreement of the patient; feeding is one of the pleasures of life.

9. The Prevention of Abdominal Distension

Bowel management

During the early period abdominal distension may be due to:

1. *Paralytic ileus caused by:*
   a. Spinal shock
   b. Retroperitoneal haematoma from a damaged lumbar spine
   c. Loss of intra-abdominal pressure owing to paralysis of the abdominal muscles
   d. Intra-abdominal injury.

2. *Bladder distension*

Paralytic ileus is a paralysis of the gut musculature. As a result, solids, liquids and gas are not absorbed properly. It is treated by resting the bowel until its motility is resumed. In cord injuries the lower bowel, from the splenic flexure of the colon to the rectum, is the most frequently involved, but during the acute stage the whole bowel and stomach may be so affected; bowel sounds are absent. This state may last for several days and until bowel motility is re-established, oral solids and liquids should be withheld, or at least severely curtailed. Intravenous fluids are administered under medical direction. A flatus tube passed gently and removed after five minutes can help in relieving lower bowel distension with gas. If vomiting or gastric dilatation occur, a naso-oesophageal tube and regular aspiration of the stomach will be required. Relief of abdominal distension alleviates, sometimes considerably, the work of the diaphragm in its descent during inspiration, and the patient feels more comfortable. Air swallowing is common and the distension it produces can be prevented by gastric aspiration.

Later abdominal distension is due usually to faecal retention. Normally the bowel motility can propel solid material as far as the rectum, but in the absence of the ability to strain, defaecation cannot be performed easily.

In high cord injuries need for a bowel action may be accompanied by signs of excessive sympathetic nervous system activity such as headache and sweating, which can be very distressing. This can be managed only by great gentleness and the judicious use of laxatives and bulk aperients. It is an important part of the nursing care to regulate this aspect. During the first weeks, the rectum should be explored daily with a well lubricated gloved finger, and any solid faeces gently hooked out. Manual evacuation is often an important method of bowel management, although in some patients who can strain a little, the bowel will empty in response to a suppository; Dulcolax suppositories are particularly useful in this respect. Purgatives and liquid paraffin should be avoided. The most useful oral agent is unprocessed bran and wheat germ in equal quantities which is obtainable from corn merchants and is cheap; one or two heaped tablespoonfuls taken every morning in milk or fruit juice produces a soft bulky

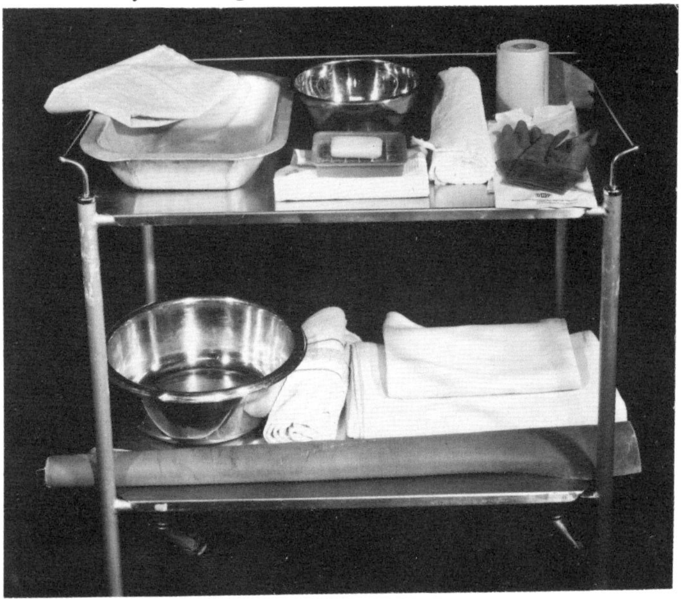

Fig. 9.1 Trolley set for manual evacuation.

Top shelf: dish for evacuated faecal material, bowl for soapy solution, soap and towel, cellulose wadding, toilet paper, rubber gloves.

Bottom shelf: bowl of warm water for washing patient, towel, clean linen as necessary, rubber sheet for protecting bed linen.

and manageable stool. When the patient is able to sit up and, in paraplegic cases, use the lavatory, gravity aids evacuation. The choice of method of bowel evacuation must be made by trial.

Manual evacuation is an embarrassing ordeal for most patients, and it should be intimated that the procedure, although not pleasant, is not disgusting; the nurse is used to it and accepts it as part of his or her work.

It is more convenient if manual evacuation can be performed in another extraction force-ventilated room, with facilities for washing, faecal disposal and clean linen at hand.

A suitable trolley set for performing manual evacuation is illustrated in Figure 9.1.

10. The Prevention of Psychological Distress

The mental distress experienced by the more enquiring patient must be enormous and, to a certain extent, unavoidable. It is the duty of all personnel to help in alleviating this burden.

The patient must feel *wanted*. The whole team must show that they are actively, although not falsely, interested in him. No chance word of impatience must reach him unless it is for his own good. He must feel secure in an environment of quiet efficient confidence for his future. His interest must be attracted by outside activities; television, wireless, books, suitable games and all forms of therapy are valuable agents in this respect, but human society is more so. Relatives and friends should be requested to visit in relays so that, especially in early days, every visiting time is utilised. Visiting hours should be very elastic. Whenever possible, reassurance and encouragement from his employers are most valuable.

Visitors should be encouraged to perform simple duties in the ward when this is practicable. In spinal injuries wards, with a mixed population of young and old patients, there must be a relaxation in the tight ward discipline common in general hospitals. And yet, a discipline must prevail; it is the senior nurse's skill which can strike a happy balance in this respect. Some achieve it easily, others find it difficult; it is very easy to sense a ward which is happy or otherwise.

Another feature contributory towards the patient's well-being is the pride taken in personal appearance. Although confined to a wheelchair or bed, men should shave and have regular haircuts. Both sexes should dress in respectable clothes so that they can look their best. Hairdressing, both for men and women, should be available.

Some degree of privacy is most desirable. Because of their relatively long stay in hospital, more cupboard and wardrobe accommodation is necessary than that provided by the average ward locker.

On a broader scale, the recreational facilities offered by the hospital require to be much more comprehensive than usual.

It must be appreciated that, as in all fields, some patients require much help in re-adjusting to their difficulties, whereas others seem to slip into a new mode of life very easily. Obviously, the latter type is easier to treat and everyone tends to congratulate him for his fortitude, whereas in fact, the frightened sensitive individual, making more fuss and demanding more attention, may be making a much greater effort. Before intolerance is shown, let this be borne in mind.

Discussion as to prognosis should be avoided and enquiries from both the patient and his relatives should be passed on to the doctor in charge. One person must control the policy of prognosis; it is very worrying if a variety of interpretations of the situation prevail. Relatives must be warned in this respect as well; one meets examples of patients being assured by their visitors that they are going to get completely well again when, in fact, this is not possible.

11. Other Complications

Myositis ossificans

New bone formation occasionally occurs in some patients. The commonest site is in the fleshy muscles around the hip joint. New bone can impede passive movement and occasionally it interfers with the ability of the patient to lie, sit or stand in comfort. When this occurs there may be a need for its excision; the main indication for its removal is the fixation of the hip joint in an unacceptable position (Fig. 11.1).

Fractures

The bones of the paralysed limbs are often rarefied and minor injuries may produce fractures, in the lower limbs especially. Common causes are falls out of bed or out of the wheelchair at times of transfer from one position to another. The fracture may be heard or felt and there is usually local deformity and swelling. Spasm may be marked but more fractures occur in flaccid lesions than in spastic ones. In patients with complete lesions, a fracture may be painless and easily missed.

Usually, fracture of a long bone is treated in a heavily-padded plaster. It is important to ensure that in placing the limb, the upper end of the cast is not levered into the flesh. The use of plaster in this instance is an exception to the rule that casts should be avoided in the management of spinal injuries. The cast should be bivalved and the limb inspected frequently by the doctor.

Systemic illness

In a patient who has no sensation, intercurrent disease manifests itself in ways different from normal. The temperature is frequently labile; this means that minor infection may cause an unusually violent pyrexia which may be hectic and associated with rigors. The onset of spasm is a common warning of something being amiss. Headaches, nausea and skin rashes seem more easily precipitated by distant pathology than in normal individuals. These systemic signs and, in fact, any abnormal sign or symptom, demand that the patient should be examined minutely from top to toe.

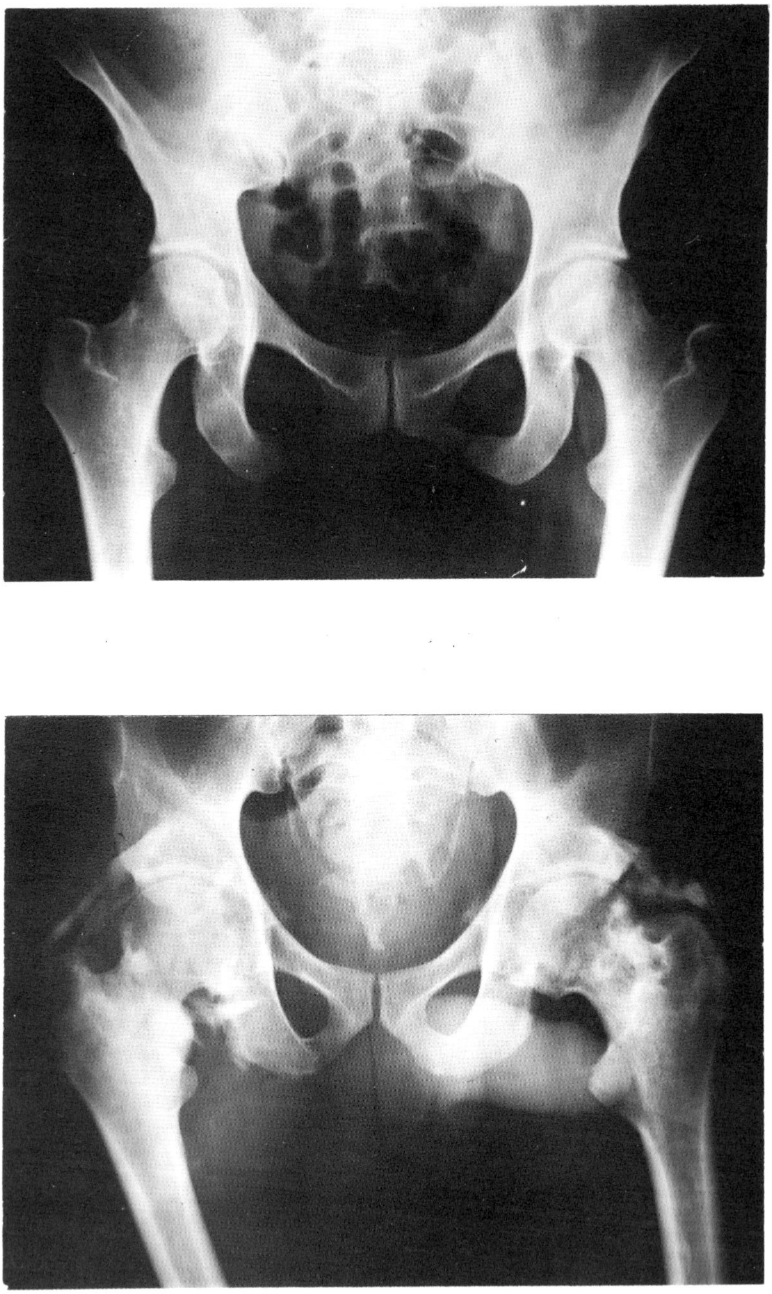

Fig. 11.1 Myositis ossificans affecting the hip joints of a paraplegic patient. The upper X-ray is of normal hips for comparison.

Deep vein thrombosis

Deep vein thrombosis is common in both paraplegic and tetraplegic patients. It is often found by the nurse or physiotherapist in the course of their daily routines and the commonest manifestation is the painless swelling of the thigh, calf and foot. Pyrexia is variable but usually present. The foot of the bed should be elevated so that venous flow is accelerated and anti-coagulants may be prescribed.

12. The Importance of Physiotherapy and Occupational Therapy

The physiotherapist provides treatment closely linked to nursing and medical care. Many of the activities and exercises she teaches have to be practised by the patient in her absence, and it is of great advantage if the nurse, in the course of her duties, understands the purpose of such measures and can encourage and applaud the patient as each new hurdle is overcome. It is very rewarding for the nurse to observe the progress to relative independence of patients whom she nursed during the acute helpless stage of their affliction.

It is essential for the nursing regime to accommodate the work of the physiotherapist—the two must co-operate harmoniously. For example, at the close of bed exercises, the physiotherapist should tidy the bed clothes and leave the bed space in proper order; on the other hand, requests for assistance in lifting a patient or in careful posturing of paralysed limbs threatened by joint stiffness or contracture should be granted readily.

In order that the nurse should understand the nature of physiotherapy in the management of paraplegia and tetraplegia, the following is a brief summary; some aspects have been discussed already, but are mentioned again here for the sake of completeness.

Respiratory management

Regular breathing and coughing exercises are essential in early cases of tetraplegia and high paraplegia; a short session lasting about five minutes is required after the two-hourly change of position. The nurse should be able to render assisted coughing and should seek instruction from the physiotherapist in this respect (Fig. 12.1).

Later, tetraplegic patients should be encouraged to assist their own coughing exercises in the manner shown in Figure 12.2, provided their arms have sufficient strength. Relatives must be taught to assist coughing when the patient is ready for discharge.

Renewed assistance from the physiotherapist may be necessary in the event of chest infection, at any time. During an episode of chest infection, changes of the patient's position may have to be varied in sequence so that postural drainage of a lung or lobe can be achieved.

Exercises during the acute stage

During the stage of spinal shock and after its recovery, the joints

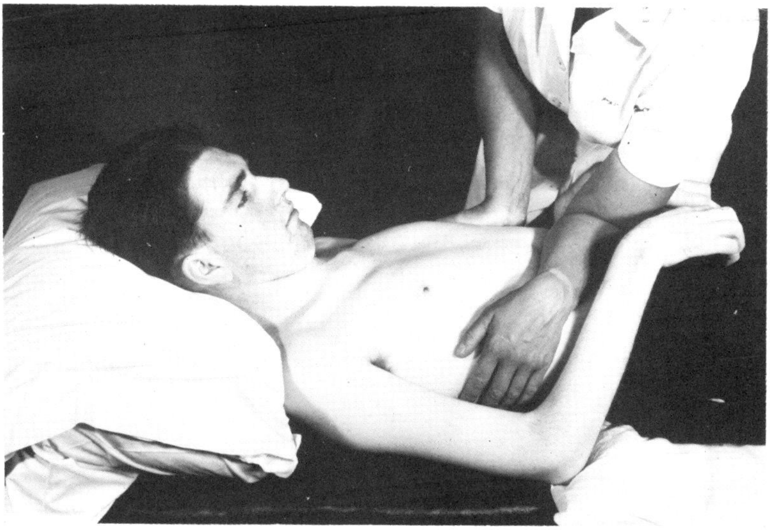

Fig. 12.1 Coughing in a patient with tetraplegia is assisted by the physiotherapist or nurse. She compresses the lower chest with her hands and the upper abdomen with her left forearm. Pressure is applied as the patient makes his own coughing effort. By tipping the bed downwards, further assistance may be afforded. Selective clearing of different parts of the lung fields is possible by turning the patient on one or other side.

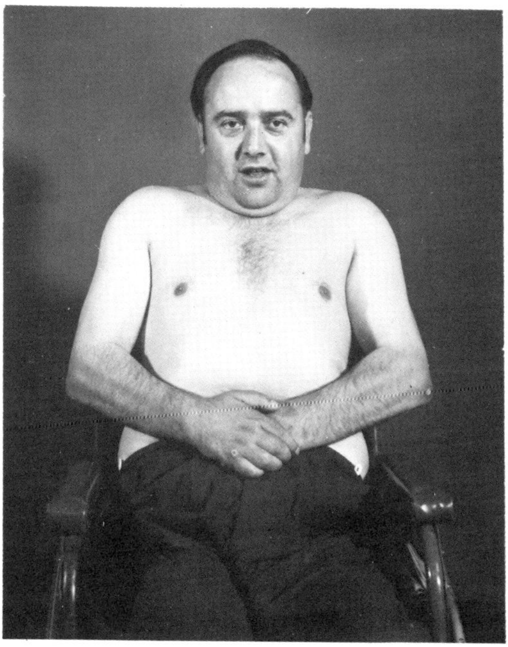

Fig. 12.2 A tetraplegic patient assisting his own coughing efforts by the use of his arms.

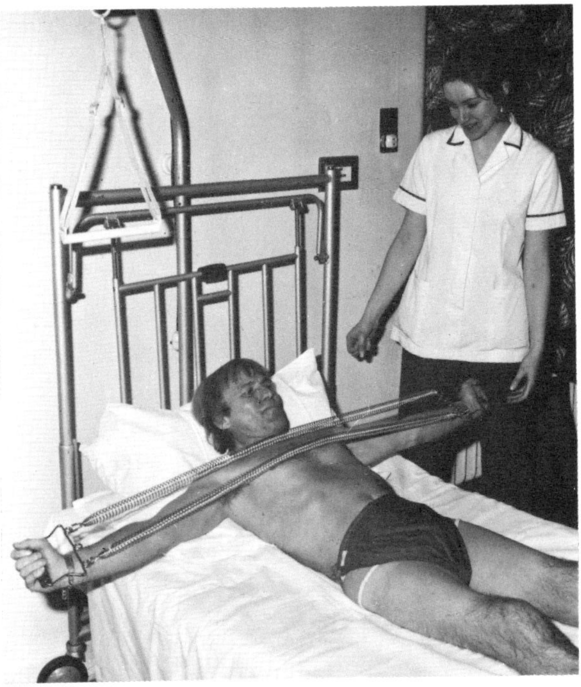

Fig. 12.3 The use of chest expanders to increase strength in the arms.

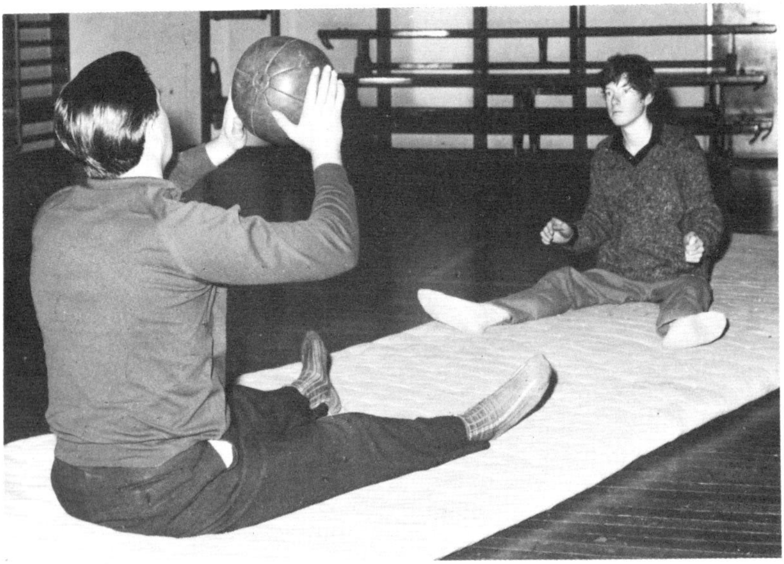

Fig. 12.4 Patients learning to balance themselves as well as strengthening their arms, by playing with a medicine ball.

of the paralysed parts must be kept supple and their full range of movement maintained by most careful passive manipulations in which every paralysed joint is exercised through its full excursion several times each day. These exercises must be done with great care and the physiotherapist is the person with the necessary skill for their performance; forceful stretching can do great harm, especially to the small joints of the fingers and toes. Without careful manipulations, contractures are inevitable and *are more difficult to undo than to prevent.*

As well as passive exercises to the paralysed parts, the normal or weak muscles above the level of the cord lesion should be actively exercised, i.e. exercised by the patient's own voluntary efforts. Later, these exercises should be as vigorous as possible in order that the best possible use can be made of what muscle power remains. The arms of the paraplegic patient are going to provide power for locomotion as well as normal manual activity and they must be strengthened accordingly. In patients troubled by spasm, exercises and other measures designed to control hampered movements must be practised.

Graduated exercise progresses from stage to stage until maximum use is made of all parts available. In performing exercises, patients require the encouragement of all personnel, especially nurses, their constant companions.

It is in physiotherapy that the patient sees most concrete evidence of any improvement.

Ambulation

The ability to move from place to place with or without a wheelchair is essential, and the ability to walk in paraplegia provides a milestone in progress. Even if not a very convenient mode of transport (a wheelchair is often simpler, less effort, and avoids the nuisance of having to wear calipers), patients should be encouraged to walk whenever possible. Apart from the benefits of exercise and the stimulating effects of weight bearing on the skeleton, the sheer ability to walk with crutches is good for morale and is often valuable in circumstances where a wheelchair cannot be used, e.g. in a friend's house where the doorways are too narrow for the chair to pass through.

The nurse should understand in principle the steps taken by the physiotherapists in teaching the paraplegic patient to walk.

As has been explained above, from the beginning the arms are strengthened by means of springs (Fig. 12.3), games with a volley ball (Fig. 12.4) and other competitive measures of which archery is almost traditional and very good (Fig. 12.5), and basket-ball in wheelchairs (Fig. 12.6).

Some patients develop very strong arms, to advantage (Fig. 12.7).

As soon as permission is given for him to sit up, the patient is taught to balance in bed using any available trunk muscles, his arms

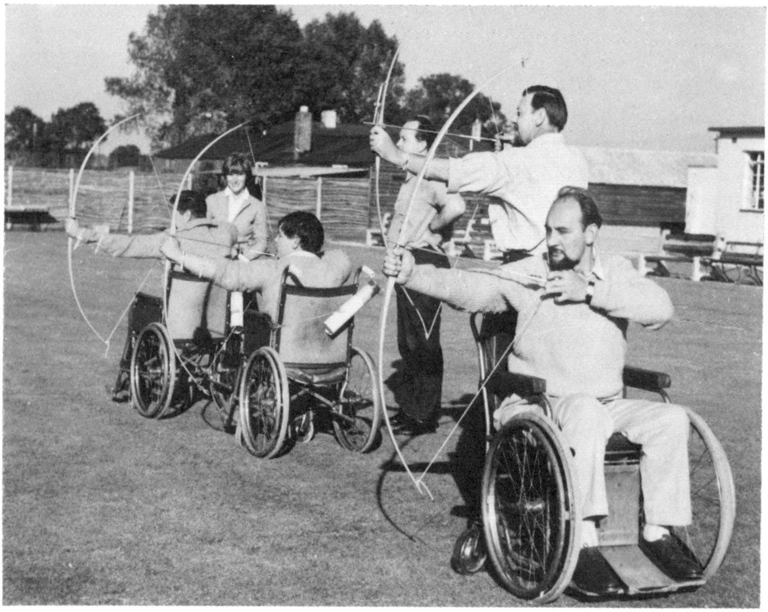

Fig. 12.5 Practising archery.

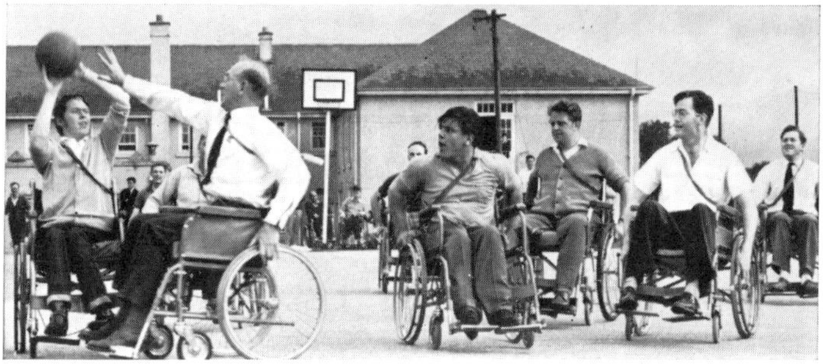

Fig. 12.6 A basket-ball match against the doctors; the patients won.

and that valuable muscle, the latissimus dorsi, which reaches down to the pelvis although being innervated by the cervical nerves (Fig. 12.8).

Later, the legs are supported at the knees and feet in some form of long leg calipers (perhaps preceded by a period in plaster of Paris backshells). The donning of calipers under trousers may require assistance; the recent use of Velcro straps has made this much more easy. In addition, the attachment of the caliper irons into the shoe should be understood. The trousers in male patients should be loose fitting and fitted with zip fasteners along the inner seams of the legs so that the caliper and, on one side, the urinal, are accommodated easily (Figs. 12.9 to 12.13). Some women prefer trousers.

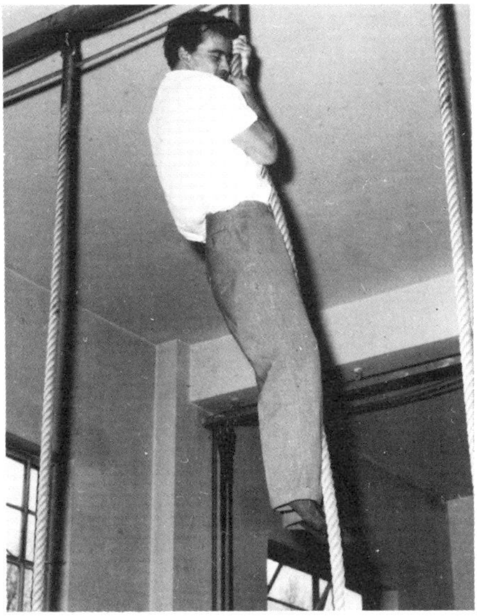

Fig. 12.7 A young vigorous patient able to climb the rope using his arms alone.

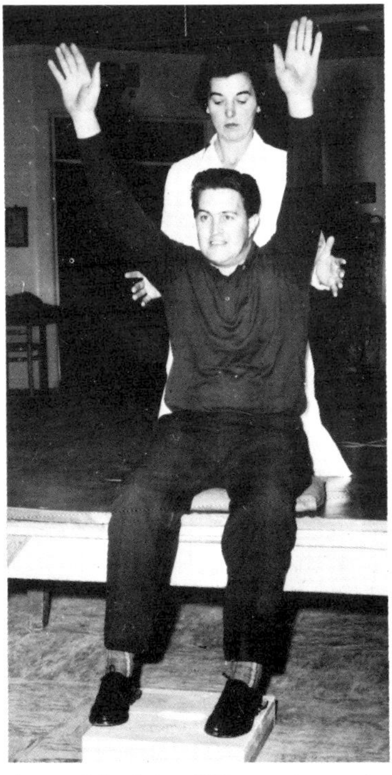

Fig. 12.8 Learning to balance while sitting. This exercise can be encouraged in bed.

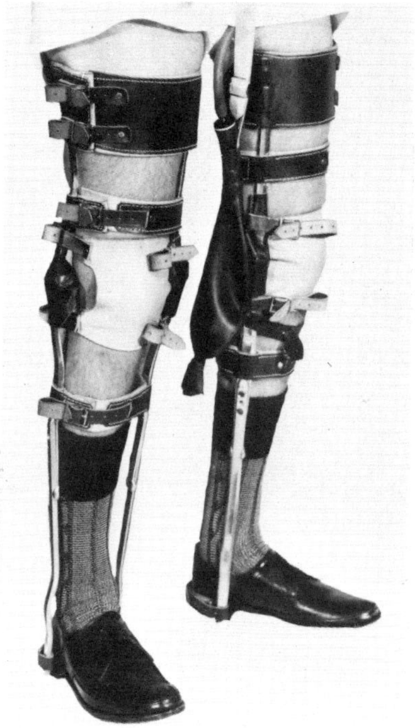

Fig. 12.9 Calipers and urinal fitted. The calipers have bucket tops—ischial-bearing calipers would be dangerous and likely to produce pressure sores.

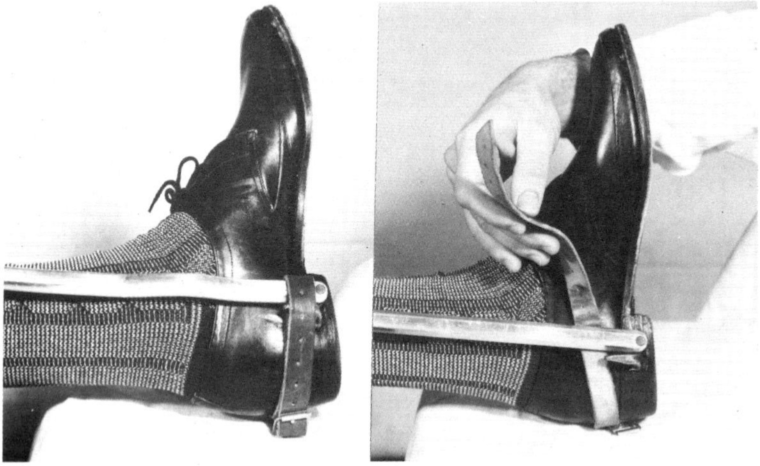

Fig. 12.10 Detail of the caliper and shoe sockets. The drop-foot stop supports the shoe in a neutral position.

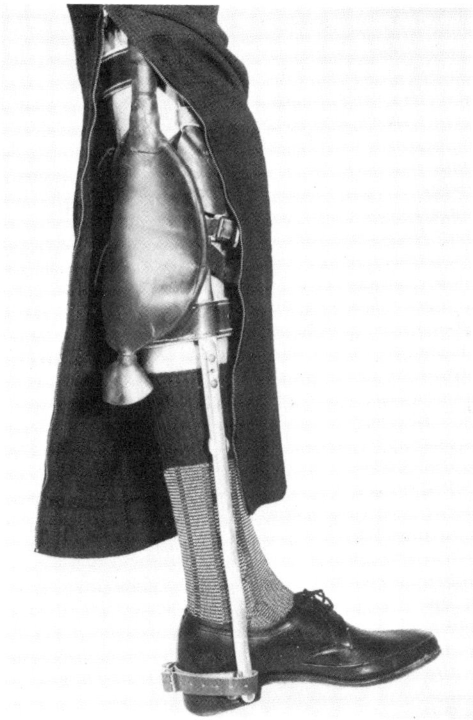

Fig. 12.11 Patient wearing calipers. Note the zip fastener on the inner seam of the trouser leg, and the urinal. Women may prefer to wear trousers since these hide the calipers well. It can be seen that the putting on of this apparatus is a complicated procedure. The nurse should understand the apparatus and be able to assist when necessary.

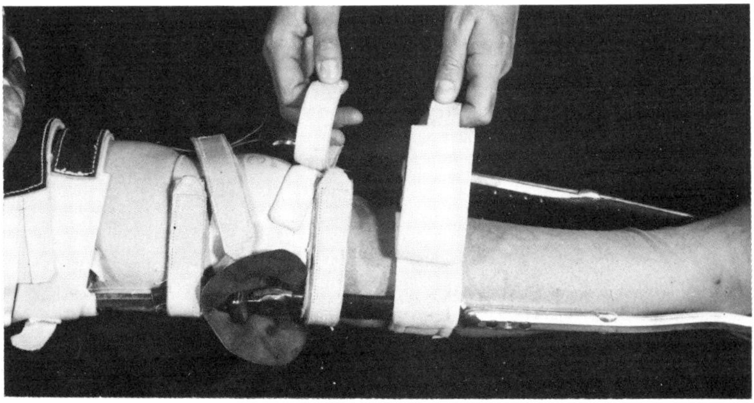

Fig. 12.12 Long caliper with easily manipulated 'Velcro' straps. Nowadays calipers can be very light, being made from aluminium alloys. The knee lock is visible; this enables the patient to sit easily with his knees bent.

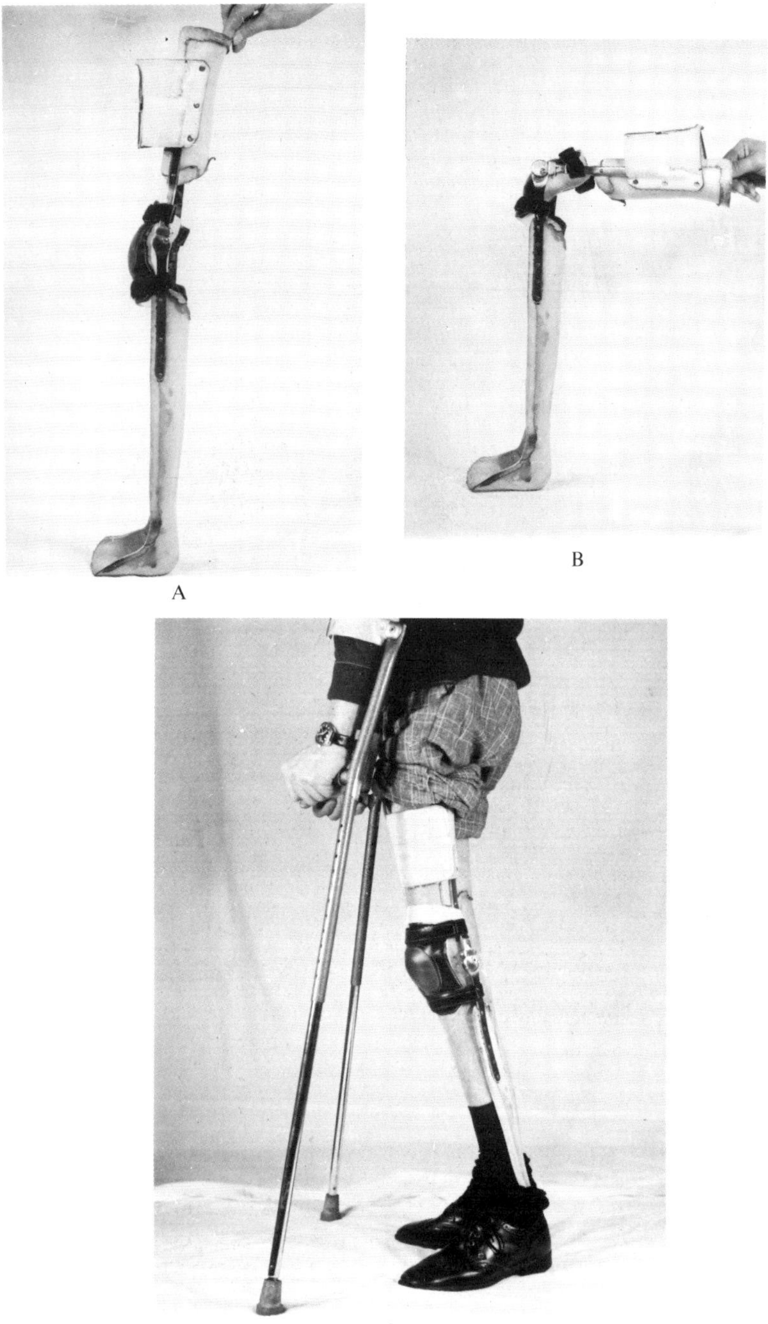

A

B

C

Fig. 12.13 A cosmetic moulded caliper only suitable for some patients. It is light weight and easy to apply. A, Caliper locked in extension; B, caliper unlocked and flexed; C, caliper being worn. It fits snugly into the patient's shoes.

With the knees supported, the patient can stand using his arms to control the tendency to fall forwards at the hip joints. At first this is done in parallel bars (Fig. 12.14), later with one crutch and the bar, then in a walking frame (Fig. 12.15) and finally with two crutches. As confidence is gained, he becomes able to ambulate unaided and safely (Fig. 12.16).

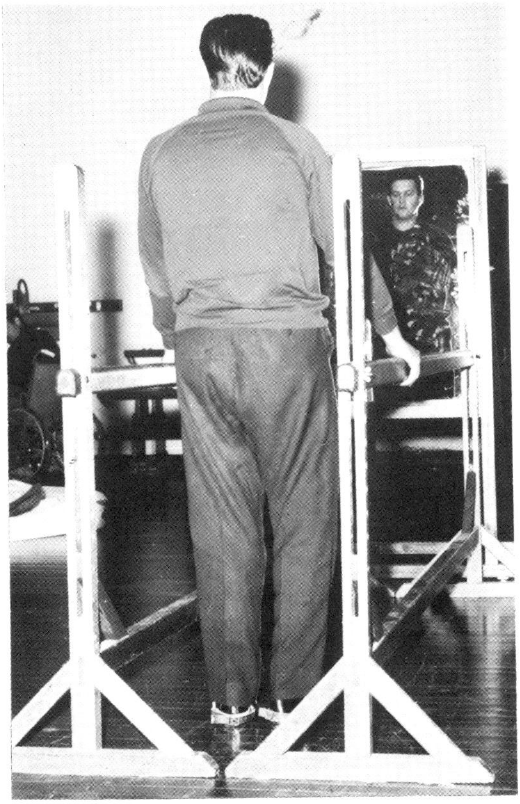

Fig. 12.14 Patient learning to stand and balance between parallel bars. He can check his posture with the aid of the mirror; lost proprioception can to some extent be replaced by this means.

The mode of gait may be by swinging both legs up to or through the crutches; alternatively, if there is adequate control of the pelvis or some power to flex the hips actively, a four-point gait is possible (i.e. the legs move alternately accompanied by a crutch at each step). Walking instruction is performed in front of a mirror so that faults can be pointed out and corrected; the patient can see himself moving and this visual sensation replaces, to some extent, the absent sensation of movement below the lesion.

Many patients can never achieve the ability to walk, and for these a wheelchair life must be accepted. Help may be required when getting in and out of the chair from the bed. Lifting to relieve pressure on the ischia is essential and nurses must see that this is performed regularly while the patient is under their surveillance; the routine is

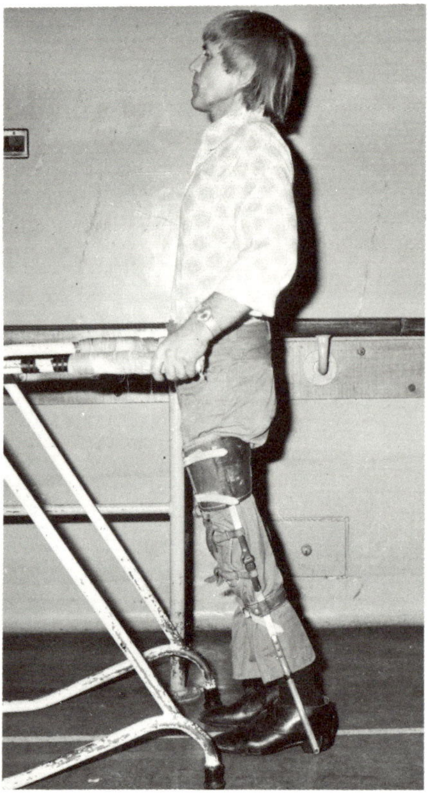

Fig. 12.15 Patient learning to walk with a frame. The presence of the device in front of him gives added confidence in preparation to using crutches which are more convenient.

15 seconds lift every 15 minutes (Fig. 12.17). In patients too weak to lift up the whole body, the weight can be relieved from either side alternately (Fig. 12.18); sometimes, such a patient can be afforded additional protection by using a battery-operated alternating pressure cushion (Fig. 12.19). The most incapacitated patients must be lifted bodily since they may be completely incapable of doing this themselves (Fig. 12.20); on the other hand, they should learn to request this service, at the routine time, from passers by.

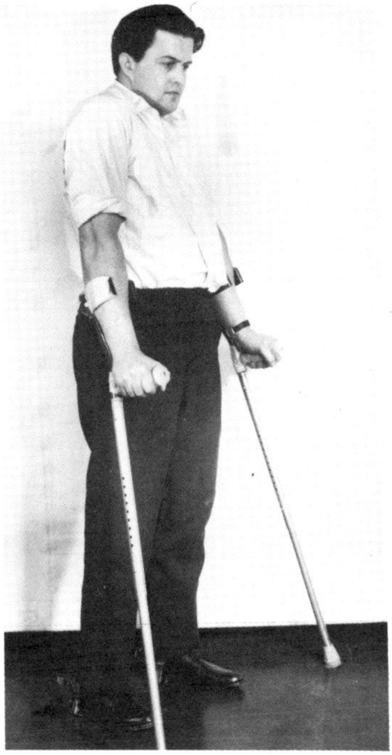

Fig. 12.16 A paraplegic patient walking with the aid of calipers and elbow crutches.

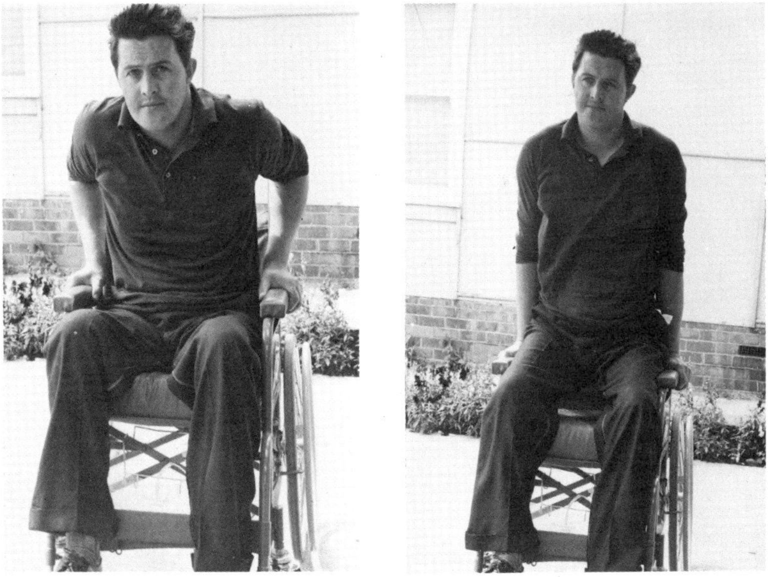

Fig. 12.17 A paraplegic patient lifting himself up so as to relieve pressure on his ischial weight-bearing areas.

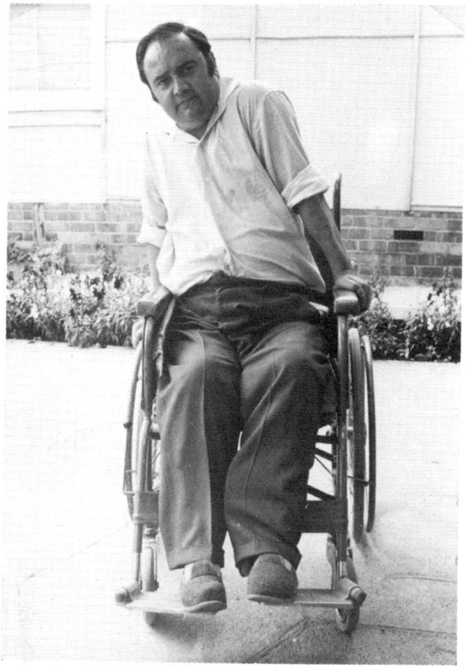

Fig. 12.18 A tetraplegic patient relieving pressure by leaning to alternate sides.

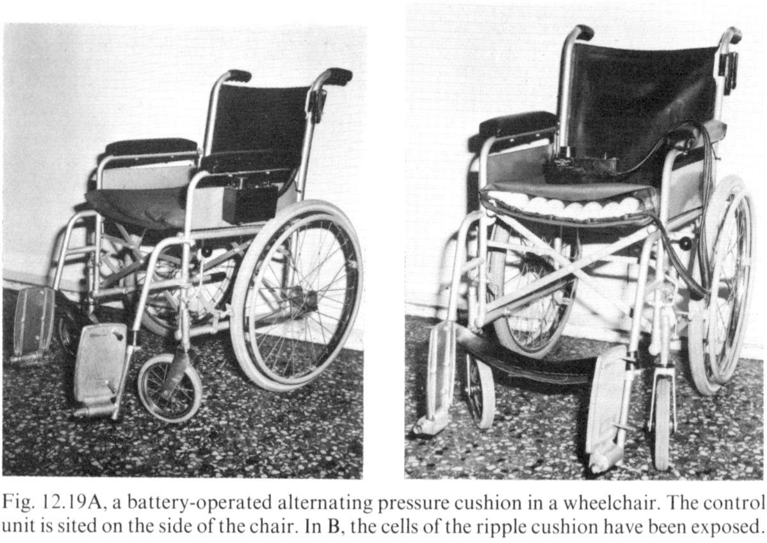

Fig. 12.19A, a battery-operated alternating pressure cushion in a wheelchair. The control unit is sited on the side of the chair. In B, the cells of the ripple cushion have been exposed.

These very disabled patients may be unable to wheel the chair from place to place and are dependent on other people for this service; just turning the chair to change a view is valuable and the nurse should enquire frequently when passing, whether this would be desired. Electrically motorised chairs may be supplied.

The hands of tetraplegic patients require care in avoiding abrasions

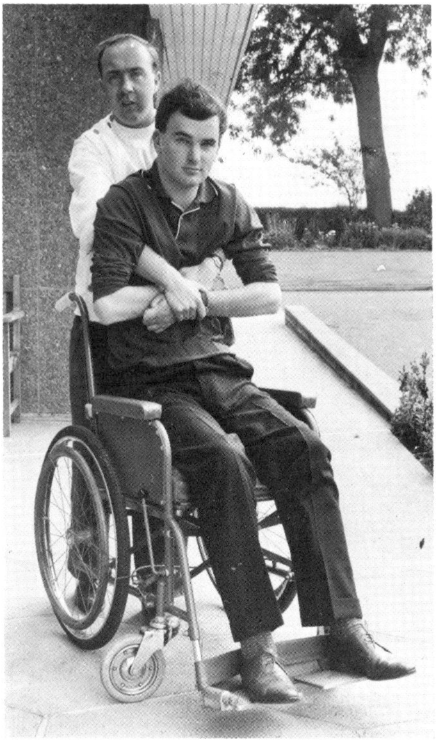

Fig. 12.20 A tetraplegic patient being lifted to relieve pressure.

to the anaesthetic skin; leather mittens are valuable in such cases when rotating the wheels of the chair (Fig. 12.21).

Many other aspects of ambulation must be taught and the physiotherapist usually keeps a valuable account of progress in these respects. For example, the ability to get from the chair to the lavatory or bath, to get in and out of a car, to manage a wheelchair or to walk on irregular ground and slopes, all present difficulties or frank hazards to some patients. Another skill of importance is to learn how to get back into the wheelchair if by mischance the individual should fall out.

There are other points for nurse and physiotherapist to watch. The cushion of the chair must be kept in good repair; straps and buckles of urinals must not encroach on weight-bearing areas. In the lavatory, a monkey chain is used by paraplegic patients as an aid to shift from a wheelchair on to the pedestal (Fig. 13.1). A pneumatic lavatory seat is sometimes advised (Fig. 13.2). Suitably sited hand rails are required. The arrangements in these respects, which will be necessary in the patients' homes, will have to be discussed with the Medical Social Worker.

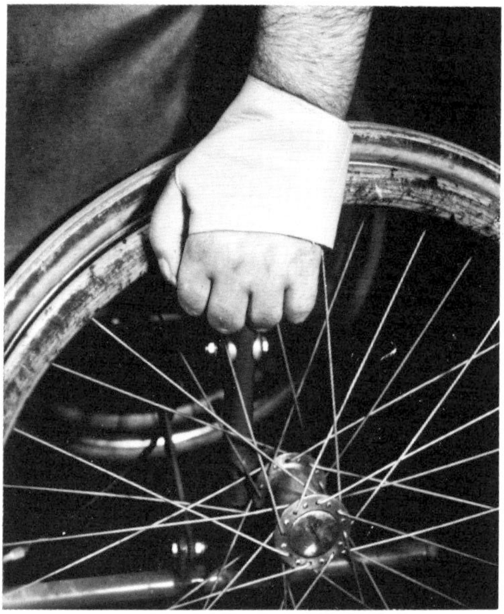

Fig. 12.21 Leather mittens for protecting the skin of anaesthetic hands from abrasion while manipulating the wheelchair.

Spasm

In the prevention and treatment of spasm, the physiotherapist plays a key part and in no facet is closer co-operation necessary between her and the nurse.

The importance of the prevention of contractures and the maintenance of a full range of joint movement have been stressed. In incomplete lesions, where spasm is more common and more troublesome, the antagonist muscles can, in some cases, be strengthened by selective exercises. For example, in flexor spasm of the lower limbs, exercises to increase the power of the extensors are performed. There are other more technical methods being investigated by workers in this field and these may prove of great value after further evaluation.

Such efforts are wasted if the nursing techniques do not support them; for example, the careful positioning of limbs as described in Chapter 5, periods lying prone as soon as healing of the vertebral lesion allows, and, of course, the avoidance of sores and urinary infection.

Other activities

In tetraplegia, the number of skills which must be taught focuses on the upper limbs, for in most complete cases walking or even standing is not possible. Such fundamental actions as turning over in bed, dressing, and other seemingly simple tasks, assume monumental difficulty, and tricks to overcome these must be taught. Without expecting him to perform the impossible, the patient should be constantly encouraged to perform as many tasks as possible himself; to do this effectively, the nurse should be aware of what activities are being practised at any particular time.

Urinals and catheter

Especially when a patient leaves the ward to attend exercise in the physiotherapy department, he must be prepared by the nurse with regard to disconnection or emptying of the closed drainage bag should he still be on continuous drainage. This must be done with a sterile technique as explained in Chapter 7. Similarly, the physiotherapist may require instruction with the management of the urinal.

Occupational therapy

The day-to-day activities which the tetraplegic patient must learn require help from various devices. These range from a simple bent spoon which might enable the patient to feed himself, to the complicated machinery of modern mechanico-medical equipment being developed at Stoke Mandeville. Many such aids are outside the scope of this book, but the nurse should understand the simpler ones designed to enable the patient to perform essential tasks such as feeding, washing, shaving, dressing, reading, writing, typing, and many other skills. These lead to attempts to learn new abilities with the hands and perhaps to a means of earning again.

Occupational therapists accumulate experience in devices and aids, and their work leads to occupation in the fullest sense of the word; this work is not to be regarded as a means of whiling away the patient's time spent in hospital; homely tasks like basket work are very beneficial in training spastic fingers.

The nurse must help the occupational therapist in her work by constantly encouraging the patient to practise in everyday life the skills he is being taught. It may take him much longer to dress himself than for the nurse to do this; similarly, self-feeding may be laborious and the impatient nurse can stuff the food down the individual's mouth much more rapidly. On the other hand, the patient cannot

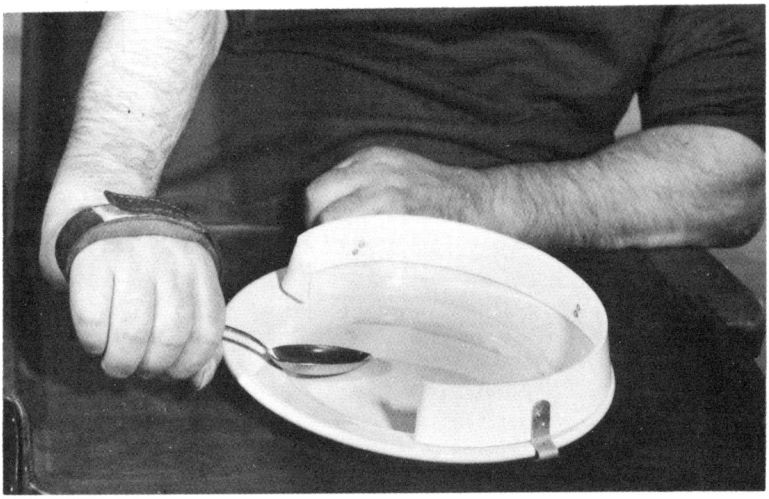

Fig. 12.22 Aid to self feeding. The spoon is strapped on to the patient's right hand; a plastic rim is fastened to the plate edge to stop food being pushed off.

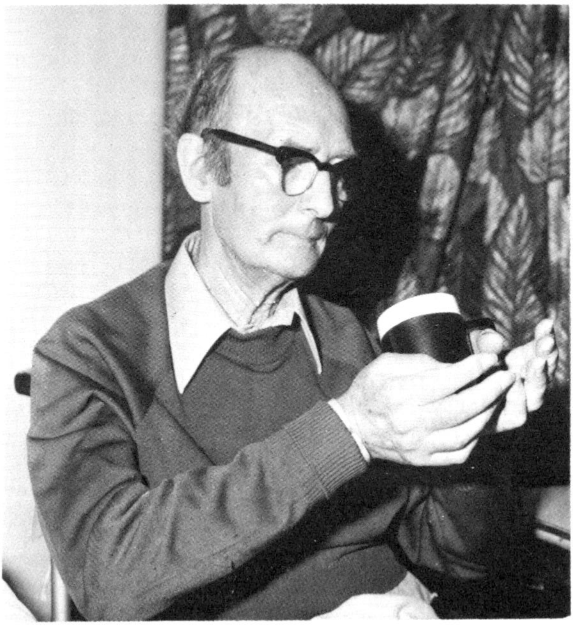

Fig. 12.23 An insulated beaker used by patients with tetraplegia likely to sustain burns.

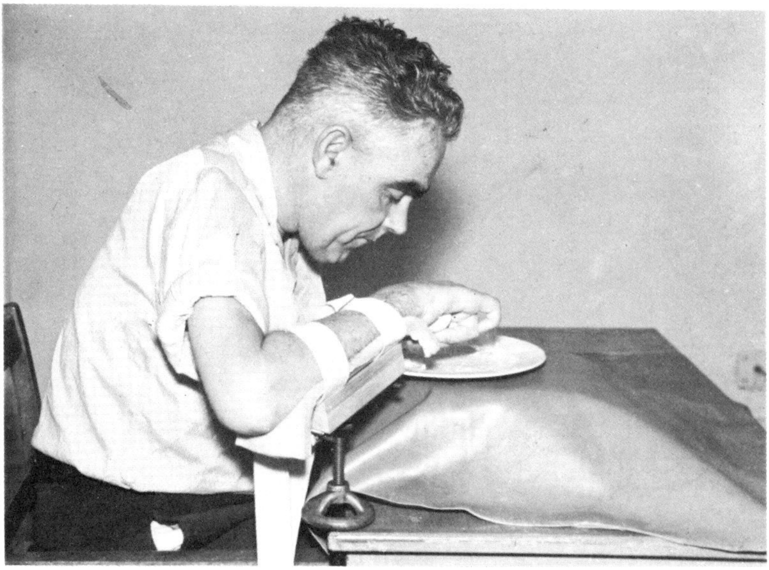

Fig. 12.24 Aid to self feeding. A balanced arm rest enabling the patient to bring a spoon up to his mouth.

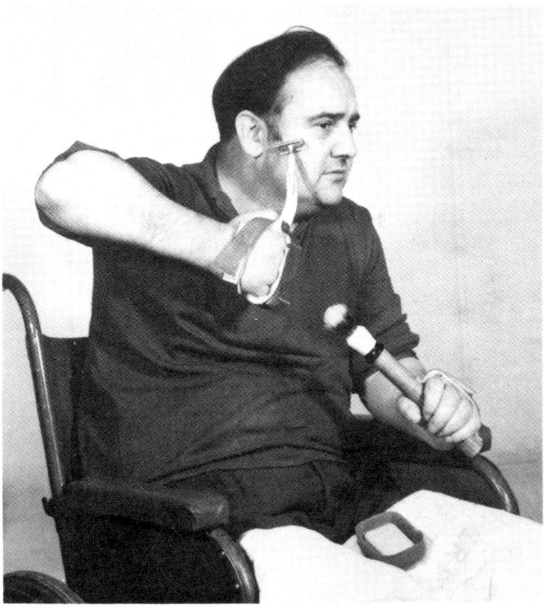

Fig. 12.25 Aid to shaving. One of the most useful devices is that of lengthening the handle of an implement.

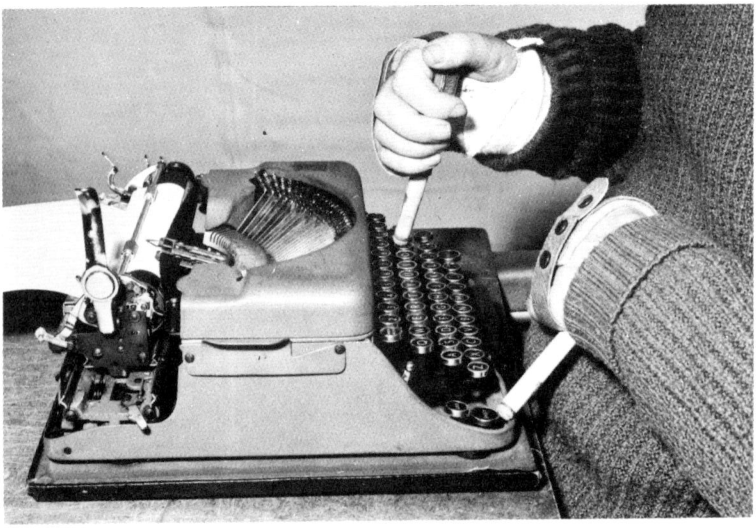

Fig. 12.26 Typing may be easier than writing, and with the aid of wooden sticks strapped to the hands, quite rapid speeds may be achieved.

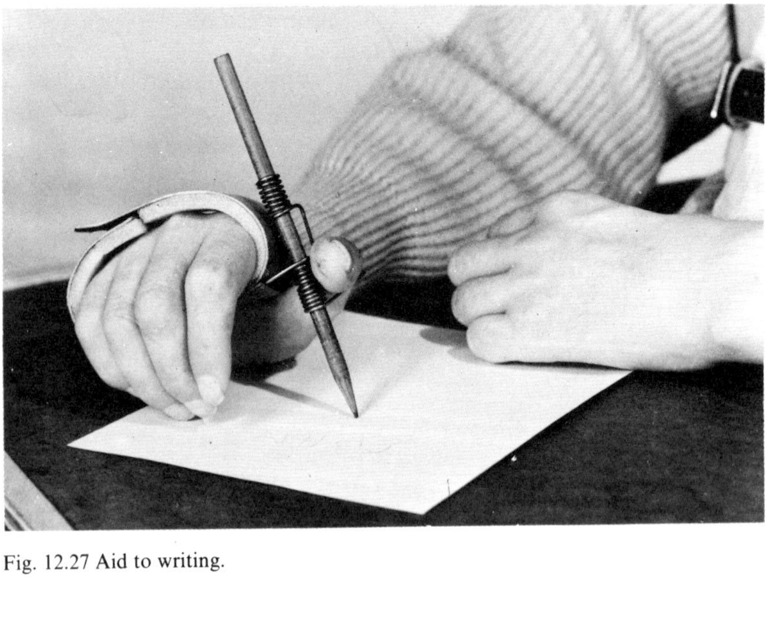

Fig. 12.27 Aid to writing.

be left just to battle on by himself, for this can be most disheartening; he or his food get cold and he loses interest and incitement; with the nurse or therapist beside him, he feels more confident and less lonely. Nursing skill lies in the balance between too much help and too little.

Some examples of the occupational therapist's devices are shown in Figures 12.22 to 12.27.

13. Preparation for Discharge

Throughout his stay in hospital, the patient should be instructed in basic nursing care which must become part of his life. The reason for such care must be explained fully and its importance stressed. Many re-admissions of paraplegic and tetraplegic patients are on account of some mishap connected with the nursing care at home. New habits must be taught so that they are performed automatically.

Obviously, the patient with a high cervical lesion is unlikely to become completely independent; he will always require help, either from relatives or in an institution. Most paraplegic patients, however, can be taught at least a wheelchair life. Many can learn to walk with their legs supported in calipers and using crutches. They should be encouraged to use this mode of ambulation as much as possible, for weight-bearing exercise is beneficial to the skeleton of the lower part of the body; calcium is kept within the bones which, in consequence, stay strong.

The tetraplegic patient must be taught to use to best advantage what muscle power and sensation he has. In occupational therapy, ways and means are found of enabling him to perform as many basic tasks in everyday life as possible, e.g. feeding, washing, writing, etc. These skills may demand great feats of ingenuity on the part of both therapist and patient.

For most patients, a change of occupation is necessary. It is desirable that work should be found for both men and women so that some sort of financial income is possible; this affords a great and valuable sense of independence.

No patient can go home, however, until he can nurse himself or, at least, be managed by his relatives, perhaps with the aid of a district nurse. In this respect, relatives may have to be taught how to perform some of the nursing care required. Ideally, they should be admitted to hospital for this purpose in order that the 24-hour cycle can be fully appreciated. Before he goes home the Medical Social Worker will have looked into the patient's housing and financial problems. Home alterations are usually necessary, for example, ramps to enable the wheelchair to negotiate steps, widening of doorways, putting up hand-rails for walking, etc.

There is an increasing group of borderline cases who, on account of the critical degree of their disability, are able to go home for variable periods but between times must return to institutional care which should cater especially for tetraplegia; this vacational system is necessary to relieve the heavy work burden of relatives and friends, incumbent while the patient is at home. The demand for hostels for tetraplegic patients is increasing; ordinary chronic sick accommodation is unsuitable, and yet nursing care is necessary.

When the patient is able to go home, the question of suitable work will be investigated by the area Resettlement Officer.

The following procedures must be fully understood by the patient before he can be allowed home safely—the nurse is concerned in all aspects of this preparation.

Turning

The skin circulation becomes more tolerant to pressure as the programme of treatment proceeds. For this reason it is often possible to lengthen the intervals between turns from 2 to 4, or even to 6 hours in certain circumstances. The duration of these intervals is only found out by accurate observation both in hospital and at home. Many patients only require one change of position at night. Some use alarm clocks and turn themselves; others, especially those with a tetraplegia, require assistance and more frequent turns.

During the day the patient must habitually lift himself to relieve the pressure on his buttocks. This 'easing' may be done several times an hour when sitting. The patient must be for ever 'sore-conscious' and daily inspect the skin of the pressure areas for redness or abrasions using a mirror to examine the areas he cannot see by direct vision: alternatively he must have the areas inspected by an attendant.

Fluid intake

Provided a discipline is used from the start, drinking 3 litres of fluid every day comes quite naturally.

Management of the urinal or other appliance

In the case of the tetraplegic male, application of the urinal may be manually impossible, and some suitable member of the family must be instructed in performing this task. The condom urinal is now widely used and its method of assembly and application was illustrated in an earlier chapter. Ileal bladder care must be practised should this method of urinary collection have been necessary.

Bowel management

The patient must be taught, whenever possible, to be independent in this respect. He may have to perform his own manual evacuation in the lavatory which must be suitably altered to make room for his chair, so that he can lift himself on to the pedestal, usually with the aid of a monkey chain (Fig. 13.1). Sometimes it is preferable to have handles fixed to the walls to facilitate these manoeuvres. Tetraplegic patients will require help, usually from the district nurse, in this

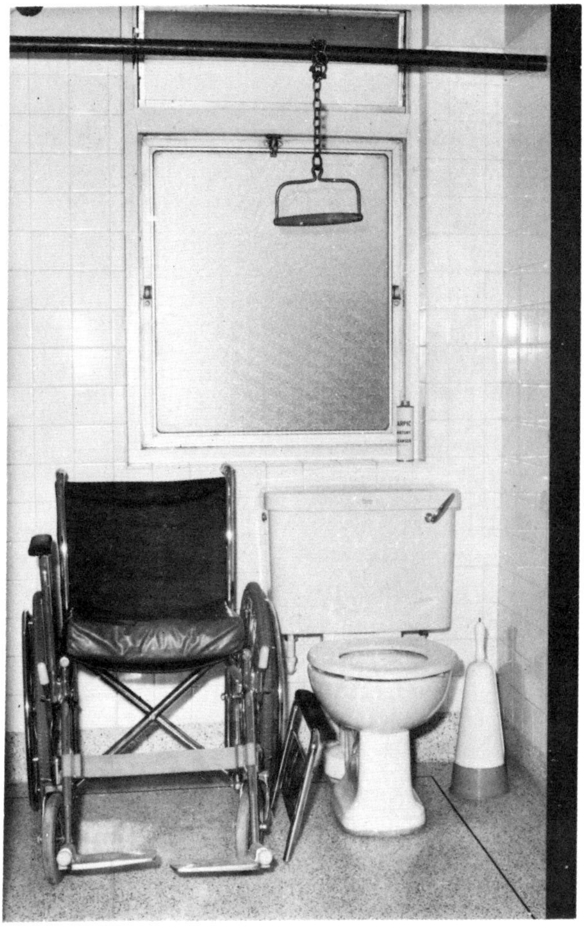

Fig. 13.1 The lavatory arrangements which enable the paraplegic and some tetraplegic patients to transfer themselves unaided from chair to pedestal. These facilities must be provided in the patient's home. The door is wide and there is a 'monkey chain' and space for the wheelchair next to the pedestal. Hand-rails may be more suitable.

matter. More fortunate individuals can function well with suppositories. A pneumatic lavatory seat suitable for use at home is shown in Figure. 13.2.

The bathroom and toilet facilities are most important, for the various aspects of hygiene will be conducted here by most patients, it is hoped. Change of housing accommodation may be essential. The bathroom

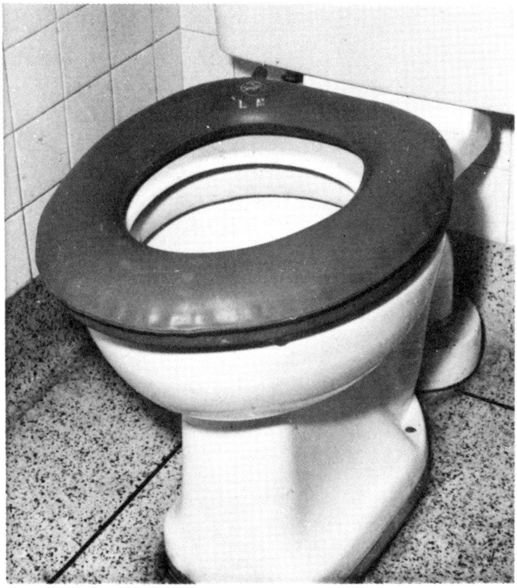

Fig. 13.2 A pneumatic lavatory seat suitable for patients performing their own manual evacuations at home. This procedure may take a considerable time and a soft seat is desirable.

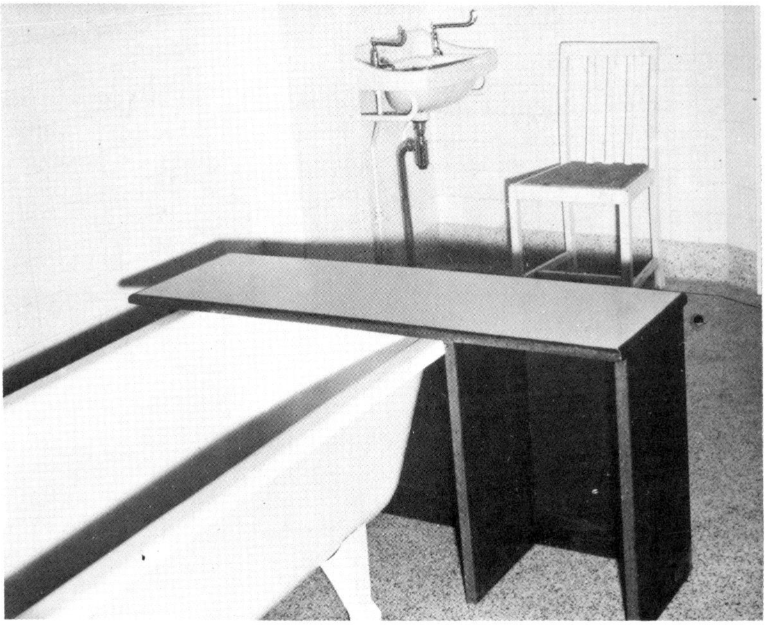

Fig. 13.3 A useful bath seat by means of which the patient can get in and out of the bath in two stages.

needs to be large. Much ingenuity may be required on the part of the patient and his helpers to arrange these details efficiently. The bath requires a thermometer at its side always and the temperature must be checked before the patient gets in. An aid to getting into the bath is shown in Figure 13.3. Some patients feel safer if they have a rubber mat in the bath. Handles should be attached to the adjacent walls as necessary. For the more disabled patient, a mechanical hoist may be supplied.

Exercise

The importance of exercise, especially walking or standing when possible, should be stressed. It is for this reason that the patient's home should have been fitted with bars and hand-rails. Parallel bars such as those used in physiotherapy departments can be supplied for the patient to use at home, perhaps in the garden.

Coughing

The tetraplegic patient should be taught to aid his own coughing efforts if he has sufficient power in the upper limbs. By pressing on the upper abdomen in the manner shown in Figure 12.1 a more forceful expiration during the cough is achieved than would result otherwise; relatives should be taught to assist coughing when necessary.

Safety in all activities

There are many hazards to which paraplegic and tetraplegic patients are exposed; a general awareness of the types of danger involved should be taught. Most of these involve risks to the anaesthetic parts and are direct extensions from routine nursing care, some examples of which are as follows:

Heat

Avoid sitting too near fires; care with cigarettes—tetraplegic patients should use a cigarette holder (Fig. 13.4).

The avoidance of hot water bottles.

Always test the temperature of bath water with a thermometer (43°C or 110°F).

Sunlight is dangerous to the paraplegic patient's legs.

Clothing

Avoid tight clothes.

Avoid holes in the socks and poorly-fitting shoes.

Careful fitting and application of calipers.

General hygiene

Keep the skin clean and dry.

Keep the nails pared most carefully.

Keep all equipment clean and in good condition.
Take pride in personal appearance.

The more disabled the patient, the less he can be left alone; warning bell-push devices are most useful in case of emergency.

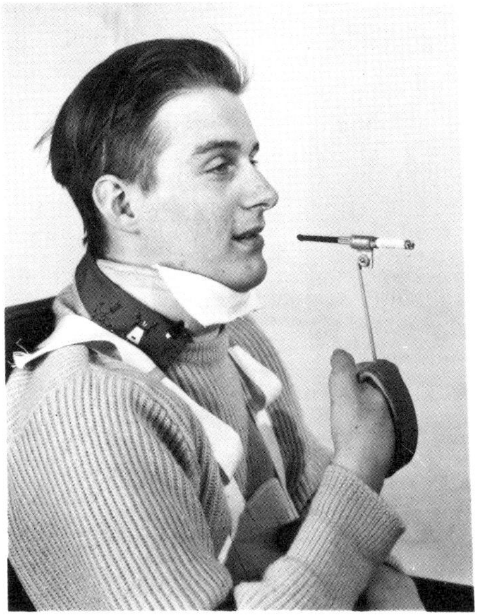

Fig. 13.4 A tetraplegic patient using a cigarette holder.

Review

Without frightening the patient, it should be made clear how important it is for routine check-ups to be performed in hospital at regular six-monthly or yearly intervals during the rest of his life. Further, it should be stressed that all abnormal symptoms should be reported to the family doctor who will have been approached in this respect by the hospital medical staff.

In spinal cord injuries there exists a spectrum of all degrees of severity. The more determined the patient is to overcome his difficulties, the more independent will he become; there are examples of incredible fortitude. On the other hand, there are individuals with less tenacity of purpose who fail to achieve even average measures of independence; sometimes such cases are coloured by compensation factors and, regrettably, the litigation may go on for years. Often, men who sustain spinal injuries are manual workers without great aptitude for mental occupation.

Patients who do not rehabilitate well are not to be despised; it is their loss that they do not have the necessary abilities to achieve independence. They must be helped to do as much as they are able, subject to the confines of their physical and mental limitations.

Index

Filmset in Hong Kong by
T.P. Graphic Arts Services
Printed in Hong Kong by
Dai Nippon Printing Co (HK) Ltd